Heart Disease Prevention And Reversal

More Than 50 World Renowned Scientists

Describe Ground-Breaking Scientific

Methods for the Natural Prevention, Cure and

Reversal of Heart Disease

By John McArthur

1

Copyright

ISBN-13:978-1495308413
ISBN-10:1495308413

Natural Health Magazine

www.naturalhealthmagazine.net

The information in this book is provided for educational and information purposes only. It is not intended to be used as medical advice or as a substitute for treatment by a doctor or healthcare provider.

The information and opinions contained in this publication are believed to be accurate based on the information available to the author. However, the contents have not been evaluated by the U.S. Food and Drug Administration and are not intended to diagnose, treat, cure or prevent disease.

The author and publisher are not responsible for the use, effectiveness or safety of any procedure or treatment mentioned in this book. The publisher is not responsible for errors and omissions.

Warning

All treatment of any medical condition (without exception) must always be done under supervision of a qualified medical professional. The fact that a substance is "natural" does not necessarily mean that it has no side effects or interaction with other medications.

Medical professionals are qualified and experienced to give advice on side effects and interactions of all types of medication.

Table of Contents

This Miracle Workhorse Needs TLC

The human heart weighs about 10 ounces (1/4 kilogram) it beats on average 100,000 times a day.

It pumps about 6 quarts (1.5 liters) of blood through 60,000 miles (100,000 kilometers) of veins. That is like 10 return trips from New York to Los Angeles every day!

During an average lifetime the heart will beat about 2.5 billion times and pump 100,000 million gallons (450,000 million liters) of blood.

It is just logical that this little miracle workhorse should get all possible help and tender loving care you can possibly give it.

"No longer can we remain secure by following the old, completely inadequate recommendations made by the American Heart Association and other so called health authorities.

Their recommendations have led to today's unhealthy, 'one-size-fits all' fat—restricted diets, which lump beneficial and detrimental fats together, along with using the ill- advised cholesterol-lowering drugs so commonly relied upon"

"What is exciting today is that we finally have the means to analyze the components in the bloodstream and improve the risk factors identified therein.

Now we can focus upon the sick or unhealthy components of the bloodstream that cause irreparable damage and, rather than cutting out the areas in which they become lodged, we can provide the blood itself with the necessary nutrients and other factors that will restore it to health."

Dr Garry E Gordon, M.D., of Payson, Arizona, co-founder of the American College of Advancement in Medicine.

Heart Disease Today

Usually, the first thing that goes through our minds when we hear the words "heart disease" are images of those gruesome and blood-spattered televised programs where they show how doctors are operating on a patient to do bypass surgery, transplant a new heart, remove plaque etc. We are bound to hear the words "high cholesterol", "blocked arteries", leading to "stroke and heart attacks" more than once a week.

Yes, I know those are frightening images and we have all the reason to be worried about that. But I believe we have alternatives as is noted below.

"Although heart disease causes half of all deaths in the United States it is one of the most preventable chronic degenerative diseases"

Our modern lifestyle of motorized transport, plentiful meat and cheese, French fries, fatty foods and working from an office chair, hamburgers, smoking, and stress, little or no exercise (the couch potato syndrome) are the usual items on the list of heart-disease-causing-culprits. And that is true. Those are the causes for increasing the risk factors of heart disease, a problem of global epidemic proportions, killing more than 7 million people on the planet every year.

In trying to stem this epidemic we are told to take the following precautionary measures that will give us longer and healthier lives:

- Change our life styles (exercise more, stress less)

- Eat a healthy diet (little or no animal products, dairy, sugar etc)

- Lower our cholesterol (by using the prescribed drugs)

We are made to believe that if you don't do that you WILL certainly contract some form of heart disease. If you are lucky enough to survive they WILL have to perform one or more of the following procedures on you:

- Angioplasty

- Bypass surgery

- Heart transplant

- Cholesterol-lowering drugs

We just blindly follow their advice, take their medications, pay for it and believe we have done our bit to prevent a heart attack.

And that is about the end of it, right? No other options, nothing else that can be done - it is "my-way-or-the-highway"? Wrong! I say there are many other ways that we can address the issue, ways that are better than what we are almost forced to believe now, and ways that are cheaper and much more effective.

For instance medical professionals tell us that cholesterol is responsible for depositing fatty substances in our arteries which causes blockages resulting in heart attacks and/or strokes. We all know (because this is what the medical professionals are telling us every day) that keeping cholesterol levels low is an important step in the prevention of a heart attack or stroke. But is it really that simple? Is it really true that high cholesterol is the culprit?

Why do our bodies actually manufacture 3,000 milligrams (an amount equal to 10 eggs!) of cholesterol every day? Oh, but I thought cholesterol only comes from what I eat. No, that is not true, your body manufactures 95% of the cholesterol in your body and what you eat contributes only 5%.

So if cholesterol is so bad for you, why does your body insist on manufacturing this malicious substance? The reason is that our bodies cannot function without it. We need cholesterol for all kinds of vital bodily functions. We will learn more about cholesterol later.

So back to my question then: Is that all we have to do? (Take the medicine and be happy) I don't think so. But is it not enough if the clever scientists do all the research and just tell us what to do? I suggest you read the rest of this book, go on this journey of discovery with me and I am sure you will also have an answer.

I am of the opinion that we should and want to know more about this disease. We should look at and consider all the options. We MUST understand before we can decide.

Dr Garry E Gordon, M.D., of Payson, Arizona, co-founder of the American College of Advancement in Medicine:

"No longer can we remain secure by following the old, completely inadequate recommendations made by the American Heart Association and other so called health authorities," says Dr. Gordon. "Their recommendations have led to today's unhealthy, 'one-size-fits all' fat-restricted diets, which lump beneficial and

detrimental fats together, along with using the ill- advised cholesterol-lowering drugs so commonly relied upon.

For those who are going to avoid dying of heart disease, it is essential to comprehend the paradigm shift toward understanding and dealing with vulnerable plaque and infection/inflammation inside the arteries, along with the development of newly recognized molecular markers for heart disease, such as C-reactive protein, fibrinogen, and homocysteine. Not only can you avoid virtually every heart attack and stroke if you have these risk factors measured and learn how to adequately control them, but if we base our treatment approaches on these new developments - using those which are most natural and with the least potential for harm _- we can actually make death from heart attacks and strokes virtually a thing of the past_."

Shocking Facts and Figures

Heart disease causes half of all deaths in the United States. The US is the country with the highest incidence of death from heart disease in the world. It is also the leading cause of death in the UK and Canada.

Globally, heart disease kills more than 7, 2 million people per year of which almost 1,000,000 live in the USA.

The American Heart Association (AHA) says in the USA:

- More than 60 million Americans currently suffer from the disease

- One person is dying from it every 33 seconds amounting to about 954,000 deaths annually or 42% of all mortalities.

- There is a heart attack every 20 seconds, and every 33 seconds somebody dies from one.

- This disease kills 52.3% women and 47.7% men.

- Every year more than 400,000 bypass operations are performed.

- Every day more than 3,000 people (more than 1,000,000 per year) receive angioplasty treatment.

The medical cost of treating heart disease or cardiovascular disease as it is also called exceeds $56 billion a year in the USA alone.

The National Cholesterol Education Program launched a new initiative in May 2001, with guidelines for a "more aggressive treatment" of people with high cholesterol levels suggesting that the use of cholesterol-lowering drugs (statins) be expanded to include 36 million Americans. That represents a 300% increase from previous criteria. Currently there are already more than 30 million people in the USA who are using statins.

Note: *Statins are a class of cholesterol-lowering drugs and go under brand names such as Zocor, Lipitor, Torvast Lipobay, Baycol, Lescol, Lescol XL, Mevacor, Altocor, Livalo, Pitava, Pravachol, Selektine, Lipostat, Crestor, Lipex and many other names. We will spend more time on the topic of statins later on in this book.*

Those recommendations are now being followed by most medical professionals in the USA. This, in spite of the fact that in August 2001, Baycol (one of the most popular statins) was withdrawn from the marketplace because it was linked to the deaths of more than 30 people and the fact that statins usually also cause many side effects, such as inflammation of the liver, and can result in serious adverse reactions when used with other drugs.

CNN reports on 8 July 2008:

Cholesterol-fighting drugs should be given to kids as young as 8!

"CHICAGO, Illinois (AP) -- For the first time, an influential doctors group is recommending that some children as young as 8 be given cholesterol-fighting drugs to ward off future heart problems.

It is the strongest guidance ever given on the issue by the American Academy of Pediatrics, which released its new guidelines Monday. The academy also recommends low-fat milk for 1-year-olds and wider cholesterol testing.

Dr. Stephen Daniels, of the academy's nutrition committee, says the new advice is based on mounting evidence showing that damage leading to heart disease, the nation's leading killer, begins early in life."

But some Health Practitioners are saying:

"Although heart disease causes half of all deaths in the United States it is one of the most preventable chronic degenerative diseases.

It now appears that the primary culprit in heart disease is not high cholesterol levels or even atherosclerosis, but "vulnerable plaque" which is estimated to cause 85% of all heart attacks and strokes.

The presence of oxidized cholesterol in the bloodstream is another major risk factor.

The risk of heart attacks and strokes can be greatly decreased through dietary changes, exercise, stress reduction, and nutritional supplementation, as well as other alternative therapies".

"The average American lifestyle, combining too little exercise, too much stress, and a diet of highly processed foods deficient in essential nutrients, has rendered this nation 's population especially vulnerable to the ravages of heart ailments".

W Lee Cowden, M.D.

I will talk more about "vulnerable plaque and oxidized cholesterol" later.

Let us just spend a few more minutes on looking at the current state of affairs.

Mainstream Heart Disease Treatment

Let's have a look what the scientists have been doing and what they are doing now to help protect us from this dreaded disease.

The clogged/blocked pipes theory

The persistent flow of blood under pressure, as described in the foreword of this book, usually keeps the veins reasonably clean from unwanted deposits.

The clogged pipe theory goes something like this: not all impurities are cleaned out and many times bits of waxy fat can trickle into and get stuck on the artery wall and oxidize, almost like butter going rancid. Once this happens, other matter starts gathering in the same place and ultimately the lump starts to calcify (consolidate) into what is commonly known as arterial plaque, causing clogging or blockage, also known as atherosclerosis (hardening of the walls of the arteries).

Until recently, scientists religiously followed the clogged/blocked pipe theory treating all heart disease as a plumbing problem and either tried to prevent clogging (mostly through prescribing cholesterol lowering drugs) or clearing it out with surgery such as balloon angioplasty or inserting a stent or bypass surgery.

They argued that in the same manner as mineral deposits restrict the flow of water through a pipe, hardened plaque obstructs the flow of blood through the veins. Therefore, all treatments were, and unfortunately still are aimed at clearing the blockages away.

Preventive Measures:

- Cholesterol-lowering drugs such as statins, to help keep arteries clear, are prescribed to the tune of many billions of dollars per year.

- Lifestyle and dietary changes are recommended.

Reactionary Measures

Surgery is performed on millions every year:

- Angioplasty - where a balloon is inserted into the artery to expand the narrowed part and a stent is then inserted and left there to keep it open or a tiny balloon is inserted into the artery and inflated to open it up. **Note:** *A stent looks like a tiny tube of chicken wire and is used to keep the passage in the artery open*

- Bypass surgery where new arteries are created from other parts of the body

- Transplants of hearts and even artificial hearts

In the USA alone more than 400,000 bypass operations are performed every year. On a daily basis more than 3,000 people (more than 1, 000,000 per year) receive angioplasty treatment in the USA alone!

Angioplasty has become a routine – performed more than 3,000 per day throughout the US, it lasts about 30 minutes and the patient can usually go home the next day. Pipe fixed patient cured, right? Wrong!

Yes, quality of life will in all likelihood improve a little from angioplasty (but that is mostly temporary); patients might breathe a bit easier and perhaps maybe even live a little bit longer. But patients are hardly cured. They are still defenseless to future blockages and coronary artery disease. The recurrence of heart attacks, angina, etc are alarmingly high in people who have received these treatments; proving that the conventional therapy is not successful to prevent further heart disease.

With these procedures (bypass and angioplasty) it is believed that the blocked pipe is fixed and the patient is cured but they have proven themselves wrong.

Only Temporary Relief

The facts are that all these measures are all just temporary solutions (stopgaps) that do not address the essential issue of curing and preventing heart disease. They still don't know who gets heart attacks and why. Current conventional treatments just follow a broad spectrum 'one-fix-for-all' approach.

The human heart is a complex organ that may suffer from many illnesses e.g. leaking valves, inflamed membranes and many more but illness of the arteries that transport blood to and from the muscle tissue of the heart generally known as coronary heart disease, is still the number one killer of both men and women in the United States, 500,000 people per year and 7,2 million globally.

Three Major Discoveries

Scientists are now saying that the "clogged-pipes model" is an idea that time has passed. It's just not that simple.

The latest theory is based on the believe that heart attacks are caused when the artery gets ruptured, resulting in the formation of a blood clot which blocks the flow of blood to the heart muscle and not so much the artery that gets blocked.

The heart then stops/dies from lack of oxygen and nutrients, in other words the pump stops pumping. After invalidating the clogged pipes model, cardiologists have now made three major discoveries:

- Heart attacks, in general occur in arteries that have little or very modest plaque blockage!

- They also discovered that the number of these incidences depend more on the kind of plaque than on the quantity!

- It is in fact the softer plaques that are more likely to rupture than the artery that is hard and calcified!

Oops!

At least they are now admitting that understanding the origin of heart disease will require much more research. They know that human hearts are not as simple as pipes and plumbing and cannot be stamped into a mold. They are also realizing that genes may play a role but at this stage they are not sure how.

One would imagine that these discoveries would have led to a different approach in treatment but don't believe that. More than 400,000 bypass surgeries and more than 1,000,000 angioplasty procedures are still performed in the USA each year and on a global scale those figures run into many millions.

Those numbers are actually increasing!

The conventional treatments for heart disease focus only on hi-tech intervention such as cholesterol-lowering drugs, bypass surgery, angioplasty and heart transplants

But lately bypass surgery and angioplasty have been called an "over-prescribed and unnecessary surgery" by many leading authorities. The chances of complication from those treatments are widespread and the costs are staggering.

Most Common Types of Heart Disease

Below is a brief description of the most common forms of heart disease.

Heart Attack:

A heart attack happens when atherosclerosis (the buildup of plaque and clogging in the arteries) occurs in the coronary arteries (the veins of the heart). This then leaves the heart with not enough oxygen-rich blood causing the affected area of the heart to die. In short that is what is causing a heart attack (also called a myocardial infarction).

Sometimes this condition leads to the heart stopping. In other words, the pump stops pumping, also called cardiac arrest, which more often than not results in death.

Apart from causing about 500,000 deaths per year in the USA, a further 1,500,000 new and recurrent cases of heart attacks also occur every year.

It happens very frequently that reduced blood flow to the heart does not give us any warning signs until the blockage is so immense that a heart attack results.

However it may appear as if a heart attack may appear out of nowhere it is usually the result of long term abusive behavior such as a poor diet and lack of exercise. Genetic inclination can also be a crucial factor.

Coronary Stenosis:

The word stenosis means constriction or narrowing. A coronary artery that is constricted or narrowed is called stenosed. The arteries/veins that are present in the heart (coronary arteries) and the heart muscle therefore become narrowed (stenosed) or clogged because of certain substances, restricting blood flow to the heart muscle.

The heart muscle does not get enough oxygen and nutrients, then a person develops angina. In actual fact what happens is that the heart's capacity to pump has been exceeded. Therefore, the cause of coronary stenosis can be summarized as the situation where atherosclerosis, the buildup of plaque and clogging in the arteries lead to heart attacks.

Angina:

Angina attacks occur in 2 forms; angina pectoris and Prinzmetal's variant angina. Angina is a serious and potentially life-threatening condition which should not be taken lightly. It is sign of heart disease! It has been described as the edge of a cliff and you need guidance (medical treatment) away from it.

Angina Pectoris

Angina pectoris is usually described as chest pain, discomfort or pressure in the chest or throat that occurs when your heart muscle does not get enough blood. When the heart muscle does not get enough oxygen it usually results in a pressure-like pain in the chest and/or, the left shoulder blade and arm, neck, jaws, or back.

The reason why there is not enough oxygen available for the heart is almost always because of narrowed arteries caused by a build-up of plaque (atherosclerosis). This usually happens when there are scratches/wounds (also called lesions) in the coronary arteries or valves of the heart. These wounds reduce the supply of oxygen rich blood to the heart muscle, causing discomfort to radiate from the throat or chest to the shoulder and in some cases, down the left arm. The pain and discomfort can be severe and usually lasts between 1 and 30 minutes.

Those angina pains are the messengers from the future! Don't ever ignore them.

Angina attacks are mostly instigated by emotional stress, extreme temperatures, heavy meals, alcohol, cigarette smoking, or physical exertion. All these are activities that demand more oxygen for the heart.

There is also a form of angina which is much more dangerous because it is not easily detected which is called "silent angina". This form of angina does not present itself with the usual discomforting factors such as chest pain, discomfort or pressure in the chest or throat. Instead people experience shortness of breath, numbness in the arm, dizziness, or other vague symptoms caused by overexertion or emotional stress.

The problem is that about 50% of all people with coronary stenosis develop silent angina and the first time they become aware of their problem is when they have a sudden heart attack.

Prinzmetal's Variant Angina

This type of angina is not related to narrowed arteries caused by a build-up of plaque (atherosclerosis) but is rather caused by a spasm of one of the coronary arteries. This spasm usually happens while a person is in a resting position e.g. lying down, sitting or at odd times during the day.

Always remember that angina is a serious warning sign that you have heart problems that you need to attend to immediately. However, remember it is not necessarily a predecessor of a heart attack as long as it is appropriately treated.

Congestive Heart Failure:

Congestive heart failure is also called cardiomyopathy and refers to the failure of the heart muscle.

What happens is that through coronary stenosis and heart attacks the heart becomes congested with blood and is seriously weakened to the point that there is not enough heart muscle left intact to pump blood out of the heart.

Congestive heart failure/cardiomyopathy is also sometimes caused by viral infections that can damage the heart muscle. Due to an increase in pressure of blood inside the heart chambers, pressure is placed on arteries and veins in the lungs. This results in fluid leaking into the lungs and the start of the cardiomyopathy process. A typical sign of congestive heart failure is shortness of breath, either with minimal exertion or even when lying down at night.

Strokes:

Some people describe strokes as a heart attack of the brain.

About 25% of the blood pumped from the heart goes to the brain. When blood flow to the brain is stopped or interrupted in any way, brain cells are deprived of oxygen and die. This is what is called a stroke.

In other words, atherosclerosis of the cerebral arteries (the veins in the brain) or a blood clot in those arteries can affect blood flow to the brain and increase the risk of stroke. That is not all. Sometimes a blood vessel that rip open and starts bleeding can cause blood to spill into the brain, damaging the brain cells and brain tissue due to lack of oxygen. Strokes have also been associated with inherited disorders, birth defects, and certain rare blood diseases. Strokes are responsible for the third highest number of deaths in the US.

In many cases a stroke results in speech impairment, limit of physical movement, or eyesight. The symptoms are dependent on the area of the brain affected by the stroke. About 500,000 Americans suffer from a stroke every year and about 66% of them become handicapped.

There are currently over two million people in the U.S. disabled by stroke.

Plaque: Primary Cause of Heart Disease

By now it must be clear that heart disease is caused by some form of clogging or blocking of arteries. It should also be clear that the scientists are not in agreement as to the exact mechanics of how the blocking or clogging leads to heart disease.

These blocking or clogging agents are generally known as plaque or atherosclerosis (hardening of the walls of the arteries).

But scientists discovered that atherosclerosis does not only happen as you grow older. In fact, it is present from birth. They found that in nearly 97% of newborn babies some degree of arterial thickening is already present! That is before they had a chance to eat, smoke or drink!

Oops!

Vulnerable Plaque

In 1998, the AHA published a study which was edited by its president, Valentin Fuster, M.D., Ph.D., Director of the Cardiovascular Institute at Mount Sinai School of Medicine, in New York City, stating that 85% of all heart attacks and strokes were due to vulnerable plaque, a 'soft' form of cholesterol, proteins, and blood cells that builds up within the arterial wall.

Plaque formation in arteries usually follows damage to the inner lining of the arteries.

The report was widely published in the conventional medical and mainstream media and actually destroyed and discredited the industry standard belief that heart disease was caused by hard arterial plaque that obstructs the artery.

But contrary to what one would expect, practitioners of conventional medicine are still focusing on the old treatments trying to fight hard arterial plaque with statins, bypass surgery and angioplasty. The result is that conventional medicine and treatments are losing the war against heart disease big time. No new treatments have been introduced as a result of this discovery. The conventional approach to treating and preventing heart disease remains incomplete resulting in needless death as well as physical harm and mutilation.

Dr Garry E, Gordon, M.D. says: *"Vulnerable plaque has come under scrutiny only very recently. Until recently, it had not usually been noticed during traditional cardiovascular diagnostic testing, because it rapidly builds up within the wall of the artery itself,* extending outwards very little. It is primarily composed of soft cholesterol and clotting proteins (rather than the more mineralized crystalline form of obstructing plaque common in atherosclerosis), which is contained by a fibrous cap that is thinner and weaker than obstructing plaque, and so is much more easily ruptured.

The body tends to respond to vulnerable plaque as an infection, sending defensive blood cells that attack and inflame the cap. The tendency to breakage that results from this is what gives vulnerable plaque its name. The interior of the plaque contains powerful coagulants that, if released into the blood, can create massive, lethal clots. This is what makes vulnerable plaque so deadly."

Dr. Gordon, goes on to say: "The discovery of vulnerable plaque and the primary role it plays in most cases of heart disease explains why there has never been a significant reduction in heart attacks or deaths in surgical patients.

"It also lends itself to a kinder, noninvasive, supplement-based protocol that can give immediate protection against heart attacks and strokes."

The Plaque Anomaly Answered:

Now that we understand what vulnerable plaque is we can also explain why some people with little or no atherosclerosis have heart attacks, while other people with almost completely blocked arteries may never experience any symptoms of heart disease.

In the past the medical professionals knew about this phenomenon but because they could not explain it they did nothing about it and kept on administering the standard treatments. In fact they have not stopped and reconsidered these standard treatments.

Now that is what I call forcing square pegs into round holes!

Dr Gordon says: *"All arterial plaques are actually thought to be the body's way of repairing damage to the arterial wall. Small tears might be caused by high blood pressure due to stress, the effects of smoking, and a number of other factors.*

The core of the plaque contains many fat-laden cells derived from white blood cells known as leukocytes, which contain a large amount of tissue factor, a powerful coagulant. This core is separated from the bloodstream by a fibrous cap. It is the integrity of the cap that determines the stability of the plaque."

Because the body tends to treat the buildup of soft cholesterol in vulnerable plaque as an infection, it releases germ-fighting blood cells that inflame the plaque and enzymes called metalloproteinases that eat away at the fibrous cap.

Vulnerable plaque is a lethal combination of powerful clotting substances stored in the artery wall and separated from the bloodstream only by the weak cap that is being attacked by the body's defense mechanism".

In laymen's terms and in summary, what Dr Gordon is saying is that:

- Firstly an artery wall gets damaged (tear/rupture)

- In response to the damage, collagen, clotting proteins, and other substances are released into the bloodstream and stick to the injured area forming plaque in order to try and repair it.

- In the process of trying to cure the damage the plaque gets inflamed.

- The inflamed plaque is easily damaged; leading to the formation of massive and lethal blood clots and a sudden heart attack.

Dr Gordon says that studies have shown that vulnerable plaque is so sensitive and defenseless that a normal heartbeat can rupture it!

A Misguided Attack against the Arteries

As I have said before; with this entire new body of knowledge one would have expected the medical establishment to change their focus from treating the arteries to treating the blood.

In other words instead of trying to clean the pipe, rather filter the water that goes into the pipe! But unfortunately they have not changed their ways; they are still using the standard surgical procedures. It is the same as saying you have a bad cough let's remove your lungs!

Dr. Gordon says. *"The focus has to be on the blood, not the blood vessel."*

Of the more than 1,000,000 angiograms which are performed in the U.S. on an annual basis, almost none of them ever expose vulnerable plaque deposits.

Dr Gordon notes that: *"angiograms can be replaced by another test using an ultra-high-speed magnetic resonance imaging (MRI) scanner that often does detect vulnerable plaque. This new test,* *necessitating more ultra-high-speed MRI machines, will certainly take the financial sting out of cardiovascular disease testing by resulting in fewer angiograms."*

Dr James Privitera, M.D., of Covina, California says: *"Darkfield microscopy, a diagnostic technique that views a patient's live blood through a special microscope as the sample is illuminated with angled halogen light, can also be used to detect clotting"*

Lately the pharmaceutical industry has begun the journey to develop patentable drugs specifically aimed to stop vulnerable plaque from rupturing – but it is still early days for them and it could take 15 to 20 years to come up with a solution.

On the other hand, while conventional medicine is just beginning to look for a solution, alternative medicine has been prescribing natural substances for over 20 years to address the issue and with fantastic results. These are natural supplements that balance the blood, remove the elements that attack and rupture vulnerable plaque, repair existing arterial lesions, and prevent their further development. More about that later.

Dr. Gordon says: "What is exciting today is that we finally have the means to analyze the components in the bloodstream and improve the risk factors identified therein.

Now we can focus upon the sick or unhealthy components of the bloodstream that cause irreparable damage and, rather than cutting out the areas in which they become lodged, we can provide the blood itself with the necessary nutrients and other factors that will restore it to health."

Inflammation (Infections): The Main Culprit

Researchers are now starting to realize that inflammation is the major culprit that can set off the formation of vulnerable plaque which is causing heart disease.

An article in the Journal of the American Medical Association shows that almost 55% of all heart attacks can be prevented by treatment with proper antibiotics. This notion is supported by an article in The Science of February 1999 which shows that Chlamydia pneumoniae (an infectious bacteria that 95% of us are exposed to during our lives), Cytomegalovirus (CMV) and herpes (common retroviruses) as well as Helicobacter pylori are closely connected with heart attacks.

In Helsinki, Finland, at the National Public Health Institute, scientists reached a similar conclusion when they found that 70% of people who suffered heart attacks also tested positive for antibodies associated with C. pneumonia.

Paul W Ewald, Professor of Biology at Amherst College, says in his book Plague Time: "The proposed link between infection and heart disease is not new, in fact, it was first theorized in the 1820s. The first evidence that Chlamydia was involved in arterial disease occurred in the 1940s".

Dr. Gordon says, "When vulnerable plaque is actively infected is when the body trying to prevent the spread of this active infection in one small part of the blood vessel system causes the blood going through this area to become hyper-coagulable and viscous, and a clot may also form, so that the blood can barely flow through that area. Left untreated, this process can eventually result in the major symptoms of heart disease and possibly death".

Inflammation (Infections) and C-Reactive Protein

A Harvard University Physicians Health Study measured and compared the levels of inflammation in 43 people who had heart attacks and 43 people who did not. They found that elevated levels of inflammation increase the risk of a heart attack by 300% and that of a stroke by 200%.

In his book "The Inflammation Syndrome" author Jack Challem says that the latest research shows that people with high levels of inflammation actually are 450% more likely to get a heart attack than people with normal levels.

The good news is that it is very easy to measure levels of inflammation through a standard blood test. Whenever our bodies get invaded by bacteria and/or harmful chemicals that cause inflammation, the liver responds by producing a substance called C-reactive protein (CRP) to fight the invasion. The bigger the threat the more CRP is produced. Blood tests can easily determine if CRP is present and at what levels.

It is important to note that CRP is almost always present in the body but the levels are of more importance than the presence; the higher the levels of the CRP the higher the level of inflammation. CRP levels which are constantly in the above normal range is a very accurate indication of chronic inflammation/infection and the increased probability of heart disease, particularly heart attack, stroke, and angina.

Furthermore, scientists found that high CRP levels can also be a very good indicator of heart disease in people who are traditionally classified as low risk.

In one study of 64 people who had "uncomplicated heart attacks", received the usual treatment and afterwards were found to be at low risk of recurring heart attacks; their CRP levels were on average 2.04 mg/dL at that time. However, some of them died of subsequent heart attacks within 13 months and it was found that the CRP levels of those who died had in the meantime increased to an average of 509 mg/dL.

During the same study they also found that in those who experienced new angina attacks, the CRP levels were on average 3.61 mg/dL compared to an average of 1.46 mg/dL among those with no further heart disease.

Since then much more research has been done and scientists can now confirm that CRP levels are "an exquisitely sensitive objective marker of inflammation" and extremely accurate in predicting the long-term prognosis for heart disease patients and people who are apparently healthy.

Dr Garry E. Gordon, M.D. says: *"Elevated levels of CRP are associated with as much as an eightfold increased risk for heart attack or stroke. Fortunately, we have many nutritional and other safe, natural strategies that will improve arterial function and lower CRP levels"*

But it is important to note that Dr. Gordon also says that patients and physicians must come to understand the importance of measuring CRP.

The obvious question is now: Should we then start taking antibiotics and anti-inflammatory drugs to prevent and reverse heart disease? The answer is no, be careful, conventional antibiotics and anti-inflammatory drugs have numerous side effects and in many cases it actually worsens the very condition we are trying to cure.

We will soon look at the best ways to fight inflammation with natural substances and diet that does not have side effects and is extremely effective in the fight against heart disease.

But let us first have a look at the cholesterol issue.

Is Cholesterol: The Villain?

When it comes to the topic of cholesterol there are wide ranging misconceptions and/or misinformation.

For instance most people think of cholesterol as a wicked substance that will block your arteries. The narrative reads something like this: We get too much cholesterol or animal fat in our diets. That is converted into plaque in our bodies which then clogs up our arteries. This blockage of the arteries prevents blood and oxygen to get through to the heart, causing a heart attack.

So the solution must then be very simple; lower the cholesterol intake and the problem will go away. Right? Wrong again. But is that not what our doctors are telling us every day? Get your cholesterol down. You are at risk of a heart attack. Change your diet and lifestyle and you will live longer. Don't eat those fatty foods coming out of animal products.

The Liver Manufactures 95% of the Cholesterol in the Body

Yes, it does and that is a fact that many people are not aware of. They believe cholesterol only comes from what you eat. I attribute this lack of knowledge to that fact that we get bombarded with the idea that cholesterol is all bad and we need to get rid of it and it has all to do with what we eat.

But the fact is, our bodies actually manufacture cholesterol; about 3,000 milligrams (an amount equal to 10 eggs) every day! The liver manufactures 95% of the cholesterol in your body and what you eat contributes only 5% according to Dr. Cowden. He also says that this new cholesterol which is manufactured by our bodies every day is mostly used to repair damaged cells and fulfill other vital functions as we will see later.

If cholesterol is so bad for you why does your body insist on manufacturing this malicious substance? The reason is that our bodies cannot function without it. We need cholesterol for all kinds of vital bodily functions. It builds our cells and is also vital in the process of manufacturing hormones.

What is Cholesterol?

Cholesterol is usually described as a soft, waxy material found among the fats (also known as lipids) in the bloodstream and it is a vital part of all our body's cells. Cholesterol is a steroid that is necessary for the maintenance of the body's cells. It plays a vital role in the manufacturing of important male and female sex hormones and steroidal hormones, including pregnenolone, testosterone, estrogen, progesterone, and cortisol. Those hormones are essential for the health of the immune system, the mineral-regulating functions of the kidneys, and the smooth running of the hormonal systems in men and women.

Therefore, the presence of cholesterol is imperative for a healthy body. In short we cannot live without cholesterol.

Cholesterol and other fats do not dissolve in the bloodstream. Therefore they have to be transported to and from the cells by carriers. These carriers are called lipoproteins and we have various types of lipoproteins the two major and most well-known ones being low-density lipoprotein (LDL) and high-density lipoprotein (HDL). See the next paragraph for more details about the various types of cholesterol.

Erroneously Low-density lipoprotein (LDL) is also called bad cholesterol and high-density lipoprotein (HDL) good cholesterol. But they are both necessary for us to stay alive so how can one be good and the other bad?

A Closer Look at the various types of Cholesterol

Cholesterol is transported in the blood on lipoproteins. The major categories of lipoproteins are very-low- density lipoprotein (VLDL), low-density lipoprotein (LDL), and high-density lipoprotein (HDL).

VLDL and LDL are responsible for conveying fats from the liver to the cells of the body. The fats are cholesterol and triglycerides.

HDL is responsible for returning fats to the liver. Elevated levels of either VLDL or LDL are linked to atherosclerosis or plaque which is seen as the primary cause of a heart attack or stroke. Hence VLDL and LDL are called "bad cholesterol" On the other hand elevated levels of HDL are associated with a lower risk of heart attack.

LDL cholesterol is usually referred to in general terms as "bad cholesterol," but in reality the most dangerous form of LDL cholesterol is called lipoprotein (a), or Lp(a). Lp(a) is also a lipoprotein but it contains a bonding agent called apolipoprotein (a). Several studies by scientists have pointed out that elevated levels of Lp(a) are a major risk factor for coronary heart disease, especially if that is combined with elevated LDL cholesterol levels.

In fact, elevated levels of Lp(a) has been shown to carry a ten times higher risk for heart disease than an elevated LDL cholesterol level. The reason is that LDL does not easily attach itself to the walls of the artery because it does not have the bonding agent that Lp(a) has.

So in summary then a low LDL cholesterol level with a high Lp(a) level carries much more risk than a high level of LDL and a high level of Lp(a).

It is therefore recommended that Lp(a) levels should be:

- below 20 mg/dL

- levels between 20 and 40 mg/dL poses a moderate risk

- above 40 mg/dL an extremely high risk for heart disease.

The current recommendations for cholesterol levels are as follows:

- Total blood Cholesterol Level below 200 mg/dL

- LDL cholesterol level lower than 130 mg/dL

- Lipoprotein(a) level lower than 30 mg/dL

- Triglyceride levels lower than 150 mg/dL

- HDL cholesterol level higher than 354 mg/dL

The scientists also go one step further and calculate the ratio between total cholesterol and HDL and also the ratio of LDL to HDL. These are called the cardiac risk factor ratios. Apparently these ratios are an indication whether cholesterol is being dropped into tissues or broken down and excreted.

It is recommended that:

- The total cholesterol-to-HDL ratio should be below 4.2

- The LDL-to-HDL ratio should be below 2.5

The current believe is that heart disease can be reduced by lowering LDL and raising HDL cholesterol levels. They reckon that for every 1% drop in the LDL cholesterol level, the risk of a heart attack drops by 2%. While for every 1% increase in HDL levels, the risk drops 3%-4%. So it is more effective to increase HDL than lowering LDL.

The problem with these ratios is that it does not take all the factors into account, those calculations doesn't use the Lp(a) or Triglyceride levels neither does it look at the CRP levels. The problem that we have is that conventional medicine stops at this point. They set the desirable levels for cholesterol and if you don't fall within acceptable ranges you are placed on cholesterol-lowering drugs; end of story (at least for them) but not for you.

Cholesterol is not the Villain - Oxidized Cholesterol is

If cholesterol from animal products is as bad as they say then why do Eskimos, who typically eat a diet laden with animal fat and blubber, have very low rates of heart disease? Or why are bears not extinct by now? Their cholesterol levels go above 300 when they are in their winter sleep!

The answer is very simple it is not high cholesterol that causes heart disease but it is oxidized cholesterol which is causing the problem.

Oxidation in the body is similar to the process that happens every day when iron rusts or when an apple goes brown after it has been cut. Many alternative physicians have been saying that oxidized cholesterol is the bad character in the story.

Dr Philip Lee Miller, M.D., founder and director of the Los Gatos Longevity Institute in California is one of those. He says: *"I'm one of those people who have been saying for 30 years that cholesterol does not cause heart disease. It's a recruit in the process, like a soldier is a recruit in a war, but it doesn't cause the war."*

Dr. Miller also agrees with the view that lowering of LDL (low-density lipoprotein) cholesterol plays a big role in preventing hardening of the arteries.

He says: *"LDL cholesterol is manufactured and secreted in the liver and is carried to the arteries in the heart the same as furniture is carried in a moving van. Once there, the cholesterol may be oxidized by the same oxygen-sparked, cell destroying process that rusts iron or turns an apple brown after its been cut. The destructive process of oxidation is literally inflammatory - it's like fire in the body. The immune system, your body's fire department, rushes "foam cells" to the area to douse the blaze. But just as firemen sometimes have to ax down a door to get into a burning building, the anti-inflammatory process can damage the lining of the artery. This roughened, injured area is a perfect foundation for the buildup of plaque, the truly evil plug that clogs arteries and triggers heart attacks".*

Dr Miller continues: *"Oxidized LDL starts an inflammatory reaction that the body tries to heal, but the healing causes more problems than it resolves. The best way to prevent this heart-hurting process, is to prevent the oxidation of LDL cholesterol. And the best way to do that, says Dr. Miller, is to make sure you get enough of the antioxidants vitamin E, vitamin C, and glutathione.*

Antioxidants work by calming unstable oxygen molecules called free radicals, which are responsible for oxidizing cells. When antioxidants neutralize free radicals, they're on a type of suicide mission. The antioxidants themselves are oxidized, or, in chemical terms, reduced.

Fortunately, the body has a system to help ensure that there are always plenty of antioxidants available. When vitamin C is oxidized, vitamin E comes to the rescue, donating some of its molecules to restore the vitamin C to its full antioxidant status. In the process, the vitamin E is reduced, but the glutathione replenishes it. That's why you need all three nutrients"

Dr Garry E. Gordon, M.D is another one who agrees with the oxidized cholesterol idea: *"The fact is that cholesterol, unless it is oxidized, is a valuable nutrient that the body has to manufacture every day in order to help build the membranes of new cells that we must continually form to replace dead and dying cells."*

Dr Richard Passwater, Ph.D., also agrees with this idea when he says: *"We've been living on cholesterol phobia for years, but nothing matters unless you prevent the oxidation of cholesterol."*

And so does Dr Cowden: *"LDL cholesterol becomes harmful only after it has been oxidized (the process of a substance combining* *with oxygen) from exposure to free-radical substances such as unstable oxygen molecules, homocysteine (an amino acid), or chlorine (from drinking chlorinated water)".*

In summary then – high cholesterol is actually a sign of inflammation. The reason is that your body produces cholesterol to fight damage to the walls of the arteries and resulting inflammation. The more inflammation and damage the more cholesterol is needed to fight it. The vicious cycle then begins when some of the cholesterol gets oxidized and then gets attacked by the white blood cells causing vulnerable plaque eventually leading to a heart attack.

I think that should be enough prove for now that the real offender in atherosclerosis is oxidized cholesterol as it can cause plaque formation on arterial walls, leading to atherosclerosis and eventually to heart attacks and strokes.

But the problem is that conventional medicine continues to ignore the distinction between oxidized and non-oxidized cholesterol. They insist on only lowering LDL, to the tune of 36 million people per year in the USA alone!

In the article Mending Broken Hearts: National Geographic - February 2007 the writer says: *"Until further research is* *completed, the several different statins on the market will remain the most prescribed class of drugs in the world, with 11.6 million prescriptions filled monthly in the U.S. alone. Pfizer's Lipitor may be the best-selling drug ever made, with 12 billion dollars in annual worldwide sales."*

"A drug that could raise functional HDL levels in humans would likely become the next multibillion-dollar blockbuster, and a few are in various stages of testing. However, the trial of a Pfizer drug called torcetrapib ended in failure. Torcetrapib had been shown, in combination with Lipitor, to raise HDL levels 44 to 66 percent with a once-a-day pill. But the increase was not necessarily in functional HDL, and the drug was also associated with elevated blood pressure. In December, when data showed a 60 percent higher death rate in patients taking torcetrapib with Lipitor than in those taking Lipitor alone, Pfizer abruptly ended the trial."

"But statins, like any drug, carry the risk of side effects: Muscle aches are a well-known effect, and periodic blood tests to check liver function are recommended".

This madness is continuing in spite of the fact that there are now overwhelming evidence that proves the serious dangers and ineffectiveness of cholesterol lowering drugs such as statins. More about this topic later.

How Does Cholesterol Get Oxidized?

Let's have a closer look at how and why cholesterol becomes oxidized.

External Causes:

Oxidized cholesterols (known as oxysterols) can enter the body and find their way into the bloodstream from one of many sources according to researcher Joseph Hattersley, M.A., of Olympia, Washington:

- Processed foods

- Various animal products

- Environmental contaminants such as chlorine, fluoride, and pesticides (like DDT),

- Air- dried powdered milk and eggs used in processed foods,

- Fast-food products.

- Gelatin preparations

- Lard (the oil) kept hot and used repeatedly to cook French fries and potato chips

Another source of oxysterols is methionine which is an essential amino acid found in:

- Red meat,

- Milk, and milk products.

Methionine is converted to homocysteine, which is usually converted to cystathionine a harmless amino acid. However if you don't have enough enzyme in your body which is essential to convert homocysteine to cystathionine, the excess homocysteine generates free radicals that produce oxysterols.

Oxysterols can also be generated from environmental pollutants and pesticides such as chlorine and fluoride usually ingested from tap water.

Internal Causes:

According to Hattersley, oxidized cholesterols can also be caused by internal factors such as:

- Infection

- Trauma and

- Emotional stress.

A heart researcher, Dr Kilmer S. McCully, M.D., suggested back in 1969 that high levels of homocysteine could deteriorate arteries and produce heart disease.

Dr McCully said: *"Put simply, the homocysteine theory suggests that heart disease is attributed to 'abnormal processing of protein in the body because of deficiencies of B vitamins in the diet'. In short,'protein intoxication' starts damaging the cells and tissues of arteries, "setting in motion the many processes that lead to loss of elasticity, hardening and calcification, and formation of blood clots within arteries."*

People with high homocysteine levels are up to three times more susceptible to heart attacks than men with low levels.

Research has also shown that Celebrex and Vioxx, two popular drugs used to treat arthritis, can increase the risk of heart attack, stroke, and other cardiovascular conditions by as much as 200%, compared to the older, generic arthritis drug naproxen.

The Inflammation Syndrome

Jack Challem is a leading and trusted nutrition and health writer widely recognized in the USA and the rest of the world. In fact he is widely known as "The Nutrition Reporter"™ with 30 years of experience writing about research and clinical experience on nutrition, vitamins, minerals, and herbs. He is the author of The Food-Mood Solution, Feed Your Genes Right, The Inflammation Syndrome, and the lead author of Syndrome X: The Complete Nutritional Program to Prevent and Reverse Insulin Resistance.

Jack is also a personal nutrition coach and has written many bestselling books and magazine articles on food and supplements.

You can visit his website at www.stopinflammation.com/ to read more about his accomplishments.

In his book The Inflammation Syndrome he discusses the topic of the role that inflammation plays in many of the common diseases of our time including heart disease, in depth. It is an easy to read book in laymen's terms that provides a detailed explanation of the damage that inflammation can cause. The book contains excellent advice on how to treat and prevent inflammation with natural supplements and diet.

Below is an extract from his book The Inflammation Syndrome where he discusses the inflammation syndrome and heart disease:

Causes

Theories describing the cause of coronary artery (heart) disease often become fashionable and then, after a number of years, unfashionable. Elevated levels of cholesterol were long seen as a major cause of heart and other cardiovascular diseases.

The cholesterol theory oversimplifies the multifactorial causes of heart disease, and is being replaced by other theories, though you could not tell that by the large numbers of cholesterol- lowering drugs prescribed.

The two best explanations involve nutritional deficiencies and inflammatory injury to artery walls, and it is likely that both processes occur simultaneously. (They are not mutually exclusive.)

One theory, proposed by Kilmer McCully, M.D., in 1969, argues that lack of certain B vitamins (chiefly folic acid and vitamin B6) disrupts a fundamental biochemical process known as methylation. As a consequence, blood levels of homocysteine increase, damaging blood vessel walls. The body's response, meant to heal the damage, actually leads to the deposition of cholesterol and other substances.

The other theory, which dates back in part to clinical work by Evan Shute, M.D., in the 1940s and research by Denham Harman, M.D., in the 1950s, argues that oxidized LDL cholesterol is swallowed by white blood cells, which become lodged in the matrix of cells in artery walls. More recent clinical research by a variety of researchers, including Ishwarlal 'Kenny' Jialal, M.D., of the University of Texas Southwestern Medical Center, Dallas, has clearly shown that oxidized but not normal LDL cholesterol is attacked and engulfed by white blood cells. What makes this research so intriguing is this: LDL is the medium through which fat-soluble nutrients such as vitamin E are carried in the blood. Oxidized LDL cholesterol is a sign of inadequate vitamin E intake (or, conversely, excessive intake of oxidized fats, such as in fried foods). Just as the B vitamins reduce homocysteine levels, so vitamin E reduces oxidation of LDL cholesterol.

How Common Is Coronary Artery (Heart) Disease?

An estimated 60 million Americans have coronary artery disease, and approximately 725,000 die each year from it, making it the leading cause of death in the United States. It is also the leading cause of death in Canada and England. Stroke accounts for another 116,000 annual deaths in the United States, with ischemic stroke (in effect, a "heart attack" in the brain) being the most common type.

The Inflammation Syndrome Connection

Research on the inflammatory nature of homocysteine and oxidized LDL cholesterol has helped establish coronary artery disease as an inflammatory process. The role of inflammation in heart disease has become better understood by the commercialization of a highly sensitive C-reactive protein (CRP) test and a shift in the medical perception of CRP. In the past high blood levels of CRP were seen as a marker of the body's inflammatory response after traumatic injury. The view today, which is more accurate, is that CRP is also a promoter of inflammation. It is a direct by-product of interleukin-6, perhaps the most inflammatory of the cytokines.

Although CRP levels reflect a general level of inflammation in the body, elevated CRP levels are a far more reliable predictor of heart disease than either cholesterol or homocysteine. People with high CRP levels are 4 times more likely to experience a heart attack than are people who have normal levels. Arterial lesions containing CRP are unstable and' highly likely to lead to breakaway fragments and clots. It is this relationship between CRP and heart disease, perhaps more than any other recent event that has raised the medical consciousness of the role of inflammation in heart disease and other diseases.

Standard Treatment

The most common treatment for coronary artery disease consists of a class of cholesterol-lowering drugs known as statins. These drugs currently include Lipitor (atorvastatin), Mevacor (lovastatin), Pravachol (pravastatin), and Zocor (simvastatin). However, elevated cholesterol is more a symptom than a cause of coronary artery disease, so these and other drugs merely alter symptoms without addressing the underlying causes. Surgical treatments such as bypass and balloon angioplasty also are used to correct blocked arteries but do not change the underlying disease process.

Nutrients That Can Help

Many nutrients inhibit the inflammatory process in blood vessel walls and provide a variety of improvements in heart function, Several B vitamins lower homocysteine levels and appear to reduce the risk of heart attack. One study, published in the November 29, 2001, New England Journal of Medicine, found that modest supplements of folic acid, vitamin B6, and vitamin 12 significantly lowered homocysteirie levels and clearly reversed coronary artery disease in heart patients. Reducing homocysteine levels eliminates a major cause of blood vessel inflammation.

As discussed in chapter 9, vitamin E supplements lower CRP levels and, several clinical trials have found, reduce the risk of heart disease and heart attack. Vitamin E also reduces the tendency of LDL cholesterol to oxidize, which in turn keeps white blood cells from attacking LDL. In addition, vitamin E prevents the stiffening of blood vessel wl1s (endothelial dysfunction), which reduces blood flow and increases the risk of heart disease. Vitamin E also turns off the gene that programs the growth of excess smooth muscle cells, which also narrows blood vessels.

The omega-3 fatty acids found in fish oils and other sources, have diverse benefits to the health, stemming in part from their anti-inflammatory and cytokine-modulating properties. Research has found that the omega-3 fatty acids can reduce heart irregularities known as cardiac arrhythmias and also can lower blood pressure. In 2001 Danish researchers reported in the American Journal of Cardiology that heart patients with extensive narrowing of blood vessels had elevated levels of CRP and had low levels of omega-3 fatty acids. Supplements of omega-3 fatty acids should always be taken with vitamin E to protect them against oxidation.

Vitamin C and the B vitamin niacin (a form of B3, which causes a temporary flushing sensation) have been found to lower cholesterol levels and to lower levels of lipoprotein (a), a cholesterol fraction that increases the risk of heart disease. In addition, magnesium plays a crucial role in heart rhythm, and supplements can sometimes reduce arrhythmias.

What Else Might Help?

It is of utmost importance to follow a diet that emphasizes nutrient density, such as the Anti-Inflammation Syndrome Diet Plan, which emphasizes fish, lean meats, and large amounts of fresh vegetables. Diets high in refined carbohydrates, sugars, and partially hydrogenated vegetable oils set the stage for insulin resistance and overweight, which increase the risk of pre- and full-blown diabetes and heart disease. Such a dietary approach, combined with anti-inflammatory nutritional supplements, also should reduce the severity of phlebitis, varicose veins, and blood pressure.

Finding some means of stress reduction or stress management is important as well. Stress raises levels of cortisol, which in turn boosts insulin levels—contributing to an increased risk of both abdominal obesity and heart disease. Removing yourself from the stress, even temporarily, can have an extraordinary effect. Consider a daily walk (which also lowers glucose and insulin levels), meditation, a hobby, recreational reading, or sightseeing as stress-reducing activities.

Inflammation Risk Factors

In his book "The Inflammation Syndrome" Jack Challem provides a quick test to determine the likelihood that you may have inflammation in your body that could need checking or addressing. Below is an adaption from his book.

Condition

- AIDS or HIV Infection 2 - points

- Asthma 2- points

- Bronchitis 2- points

- Celiac Disease or Gluten Intolerance 2- points

- Coronary Artery (Heart) Disease 2- points

- Diabetes or Elevated Blood Sugar 2- points

- Gingivitis or Periondontitis (Gum Disease) 2- points

- Hepatitis 2- points

- Inflammatory Bowel Disease 2- points

- Rheumatoid Arthritis 2- points

- Osteoarthritis 2- points

- Eczema, Psoriasis or Frequent Sunburn 2- points

- Stomach Ulcers 2- points

- Ulcerated Varicose Veins 2- points

- Obese (overweight by more than 20 pounds) (8 * kg) carrying that extra fat mostly around your waste 2- points

- Smoke or chew tobacco 2- points

- Recent Physical Injury (sport, accident or other) 1- point

- Consistent Stiff or Aching Joints (including fingers) 1- point

- Body Feels Stiff when getting out of bed in the morning 1- point

- Overweight by more than 10 pounds (4kg) carrying that extra fat mostly around your waste 1- point

- Nose stuffed or runny all the time 1- point

- Regular injuries and bruises during the year as part of work or sport 1- point

- Surgery recently 1- point

- Frequent Colds and Flu 1- point

- Seasonal Allergies from pollen or mold 1- point

- Skin sores or rashes that does not go away or take a very long time to heal 1- point

Interpretation

- **Score 0-1** – Low or no Inflammation

- **Score 2-6** - Moderate Inflammation. Your long term health could be at risk.

- **Score 7-20** - High Inflammation. Requires immediate attention.

- **Score 21+** - Very High Inflammation. Requires immediate attention.

Cholesterol and Genes

In most cases, high cholesterol and triglycerides are the consequence of lifestyle and diet. However, in 1 out of 500 people the problem is caused by genetic factors.

According to Dr Robert A. Anderson, M.D. founding President of the American Board of Holistic Medicine, there are occurrences of rare but severe inherited cholesterol metabolism issues.

Dr Anderson says: *"In such cases, male family members are prone to heart attacks as early as their twenties.*

Hyperhomocysteinemia, a condition characterized by poor metabolism of the amino acids methionine and cysteine, is a more common, yet less severe genetic risk factor, although some researchers believe that it may account for 20% of heart attacks and strokes. Elevated blood fibrinogen levels, another serious risk factor for heart disease, can also be influenced by heredity".

As we age we are also more vulnerable to diseases like diabetes. Cholesterol levels are likely to rise in people with diabetes and also in people as they age.

Fortunately, the same steps for lowering your cholesterol levels discussed in the later parts of this book will benefit those with inherited high cholesterol, diabetes and aging.

Other Heart Disease Risk factors

There are also a number of additional factors and conditions that increase the risk of heart disease such as:

- Hypertension (high blood pressure)

- Diabetes and Insulin Resistance

- Hypothyroidism (underactive thyroid)

- Smoking

- Mercury Poisoning

- Gum disease and other Oral Diseases

- Nutritional deficiencies (especially coenzyme Q10, magnesium, and selenium)

Hypertension (high blood pressure)

High blood pressure causes damage to the arteries and if not treated increases the risk of heart disease dramatically. The problem of hypertension is not detected easily and many people are not aware of the fact that they have high blood pressure until they are being tested.

The current guidelines for high blood pressure are as follows:

- **High normal pressure**: 130-139/85-89

- **Stage 1 hypertension**: 140-159/90-99

- **Stage 2 hypertension**: 160-179/100-109

- **Stage 3 hypertension**: 180-209/110-119

Dr Robert A. Anderson, M.D. says: *"Approximately 95% of hypertension is labeled by conventional doctors as "essential" or cause unknown. However, a large percentage of these hypertensive patients have nutritional deficiencies, heavy metal toxicity (especially lead, mercury; nickel, and cadmium), toxicity from pesticides and chemical poisons, or marked autonomic nervous system imbalance. When these issues are corrected, the hypertension usually dramatically improves or resolves".*

Diabetes and Insulin Resistance

The role that diabetes play in heart disease has been known for almost 50 years now, especially Type II (adult-onset) diabetes.

Dr. Anderson says: *"The presence of diabetes accelerates premature degeneration of arterial walls, inducing circulatory deficiencies."*

Type II diabetes can also cause a number of biochemical changes, including increased levels of corticosteroids, increased biochemical stress, and the production of high levels of free radicals.

Insulin resistance which is also sometimes referred to as syndrome X is regarded as the precursor to Type II diabetes also plays a significant role in heart disease, in particular in families which are prone to heart disease.

Researchers found that the incidence of insulin resistance blood-vessel blockage at an early age (55 for men, 65 for women) is common place. They also found that people with insulin resistance that attract heart disease almost always have higher insulin levels, higher triglycerides, higher fibrinogen, and lower HDL cholesterol, compared to their family members who don't have heart disease.

Hypothyroidism (underactive thyroid)

An underactive thyroid is another one that contributes to heart disease but at the same time it is one of those crucial risk factors that are easily overlooked by the conventional practitioners.

Dr Broda O. Barnes, M.D., a Connecticut physician who is specializing in the identification and treatment of disease conditions associated with low thyroid activity demonstrated the relationship between hypothyroidism and heart disease with a study of 1,569 patients, grouped according to six categories of age or heart status.

His findings were as follows:

- As a frame of reference, he used the Framingham Heart Study which tracked the health status of thousands of men and women over several decades since 1949.

- He found that among women 30-59 years old, while there were 7.6 expected coronary cases according to the Framingham results (where no thyroid treatment was given), among his thyroid—treated patients there were no cases.

- Similarly, for those women with high risk of heart disease, Framingham results predicted 7.3 cases, but among Dr. Barnes's patients there were none.

- For women over 60, Framingham predicted 7.8 cases; Dr. Barnes's group had none.

- For men ages 30-59, the ratio was 12.8 (Framingham) to 1 (Barnes);

- for high-risk males, it was 18.5 to 2;

- and for men 60 and over, it was 18 to 1.

In summary, out of an equivalent patient population, Framingham results expected 72 coronary cases, but among Dr. Barnes's thyroid-treated patients, there were only four cases.

Other researchers have also shown that people with an underactive thyroid have higher levels of LDL cholesterol and are more like to have heart disease. In fact the latest research actually shows that the problem is much bigger than what was generally believed up till now, when they found that people with very mild cases of hypothyroidism have significantly higher levels of LDL cholesterol and lipoprotein (a).

Therefore it is extremely important to make sure that your high cholesterol levels are not perhaps caused by hypothyroidism.

Smoking

More people are dying from heart attacks because of smoking than from cancer caused by smoking. It is estimated that in the USA about 191,000 people per year die from heart diseases which is directly related to smoking this is about 44% more than people dying from cancer related to smoking.

According to the American Heart Association a further ± 40,000 attracts heart disease because of second hand smoking. Research found that regular exposure to secondary smoke nearly doubles the risk of heart attack and death in non-smokers.

Dr. Ichiro Kawachi of the Harvard School of Public Health says:

"The 4,000 chemicals in tobacco smoke just about do everything that we know that is harmful to the heart. They will damage the lining of the arteries, increase the stickiness of your blood, and therefore increase the chances that you will develop clotting and a heart attack."

Mercury Poisoning

Mercury is another one of those culprits. The big problem is that mercury poisoning is a hidden cause of heart disease that very few people know about. Alternative medicine practitioners know about this and usually test for the presence of heavy metals including mercury.

The most common cause of mercury poisoning is introduced through dental fillings, but can also be caused by various vaccines, as well as exposure to mercury in the environment and from certain fish.

In 1974, Russian researchers first discovered that when rabbits were exposed to mercury vapor, it inactivated enzymes necessary for heart muscle contraction. Other research shows that mercury seems to interfere with the normal processing of nutrients that supply arterial smooth muscle, leading to it becoming inflexible.

Mercury seems to obstruct the manufacturing of cholesterol from arterial cell walls and depositing of cholesterol in the liver for removal from the body. Because it interferes with the process of fat removing it may be contributing to the high total cholesterol. Therefore it is important that whenever there is an unexplained elevation of cholesterol, a check for mercury toxicity should be performed.

Dr. Cowden goes as far as recommending that all people with coronary disease should have all the mercury containing fillings removed from their teeth because it not only raises cholesterol levels, but it can also leak out and interfere with the nerve bundles in the heart muscle. He says: *"Because the mercury was poisoning those ganglia, or nerve bundles, the patient's heart started having problems, such as impaired blood supply or disturbed heart rhythm,"* he says. *"When we got the mercury out of their teeth, then used chelating agents to get the mercury out of their body tissues, the heart problems cleared up and they were able to discontinue their heart medications for arrhythmia and angina."*

Gum Disease and Other Oral Disease

Another little secret is that gum and oral disease could also have a relationship to heart disease, especially stroke.

During a study of 10,000 people it was found that strokes are significantly more prevalent amongst people with gum disease (periodontitis). Researchers found that the bacteria associated with gum disease enter the bloodstream, damaging the lining of blood vessels and stimulating clotting.

The study's lead researcher advised: *"People may need to pay more attention to their oral health, as it may influence their systemic health."*

Dangers of Conventional Heart Disease Treatment

Cholesterol-Lowering Drugs

The traditional treatment for high cholesterol is to try and lower the levels through the prescription of cholesterol-lowering drugs. The prescription of statins is by far the most popular of the cholesterol-lowering drugs mainly because of the aggressive marketing by drug companies.

More than 30 million statin prescriptions per year are being dished out in the USA in spite of the fact that it is not high cholesterol but rather the levels of oxidized cholesterol that causes heart disease.

Side Effects of Conventional Cholesterol Lowering Drugs

The most worrying factor however about this trend is that research has proved the serious side effects and ineffectiveness that statins have on the human body as shown by various studies and researchers.

For instance:

- In some studies it has been found that the drugs used to lower LDL cholesterol actually raise it in people who already have the highest levels!

- A study conducted in Finland reported that deaths from heart attacks and strokes were 46% higher in those taking cholesterol-lowering drugs!

- Even newer drugs believed to be safer also have damaging side effects, for instance lovastatin lowers the blood levels of coenzyme Q10, a vital antioxidant that helps the body resist heart damage.

No major study to date could prove that the use of cholesterol lowering drugs actually extend a person's life span. In fact many of these studies have shown that the use of these drugs actually increases the death rate for non-cardiovascular mortality. In other words while these drugs reduced the number of deaths from heart attacks and strokes, they increased the overall death rate!

Conventional Cholesterol Lowering Drugs

Researchers found that cholesterol-lowering drugs may increase overall mortality rate because it is in fact toxic to the liver and extremely carcinogenic (cancer-causing). The Journal of the American, Medical Association (JAMA) summarized the findings of a number of studies on the cancer causing properties of cholesterol-lowering drugs which proved beyond any doubt the risks of getting cancer when using these drugs. The article also proved that the risks carried by these drugs are far above FDA guidelines.

The article asked several questions and provide answers that were extremely interesting. Here is an example:

How did it happen that cholesterol-lowering drugs were approved by the FDA for long-term use in spite of their animal carcinogenicity? To address the question, we obtained minutes of the Endocrinologic and Metabolic Drugs Advisory Committee meetings (under the Freedom of Information Act) at which lovastatin and gemfibrozil—the two most popular cholesterol-lowering drugs—were discussed.... . The only reported discussion of animal carcinogenicity studies at the FDA advisory committee meeting on lovastatin (February 19 and 20, 1987) was by a representative of Merck Sharp & Dohme (makers of the Mevacor brand of lovastatin), who downplayed the importance of the studies.

The minutes from the meeting on gemfibrozil (October 17, 1988) are extremely enlightening. The committee did discuss the carcinogenicity of the drug. The minutes state:

Dr. Troendle [deputy director, Division of Metabolism and Endocrine Drug Products for the FDA] noted that gemfibrozil belongs to a class of drugs that has been shown to increase total mortality. It has been shown to have animal carcinogenicity, and she does not believe the FDA has ever approved a drug for long-term prophylactic use that was carcinogenic at such low multiples of the human dose as gemfibrozil.

At the end of the meeting members were asked to vote and it turned out that only 3 of the 9 members of the advisory committee believed the potential benefit of gemfibrozil outweighed the risk.

The big shock came when the FDA decided to ignore the committee's recommendation and grant approval for the gemfibrozil drug. Lopid (gemfibrozil) is now the second most popular cholesterol-lowering drug, behind Mevacor (lovastatin) in the world!

The authors of this article strongly advised against the use of cholesterol-lowering drug treatment but the widespread use of these drugs ignores this recommendation.

Dangers of using Statin Drugs

Below is my summary of an article by Sally Fallon and Mary G. Enig, PhD titled: **Dangers of Statin Drugs: What You Haven't Been Told About Popular Cholesterol-Lowering Medicines.**

You can read the full article at the website below. www.westonaprice.org/moderndiseases/statin.html

They (Sally Fallon and Mary G. Enig) call hypercholesterolemia (high cholesterol) the health issue of the 21st century but also at the same time call it an "invented" disease. Because it only became a "problem" since physicians learned how to measure blood cholesterol levels. Furthermore they argue that high cholesterol does not have outward symptoms like other illnesses that make you feel bad. So part of the issue is that those physicians have to tell people who actually feel good that they are in fact sick!

Over the past 25-30 years the medical community has moved the goals posts of what is being seen as high cholesterol from 240 mg/dl to 200 mg/dl and now 180 mg/dl – always lower.

How Statins Work

Statins works by inhibiting the formation of certain enzymes in the body and that is where the potential for numerous side effects lies, because statins inhibit not only the formation of cholesterol, but a whole range of other substances many of which are vital for the biochemical functions of our body. They go on to explain that cholesterol is one of three end products in the body of which ubiquinone (known as Co-Enzyme Q10) is critical for cellular nutrition. The heart requires high levels of Co-Q10 and is found in all cell membranes where it plays a role in maintaining membrane integrity so critical to nerve conduction and muscle integrity.

Side effects of Co-Q10 deficiency include muscle wasting leading to weakness and severe back pain, heart failure (because the heart is a muscle!), neuropathy and inflammation of the tendons and ligaments, often leading to rupture.

The Role of Cholesterol in our Bodies

Statins inhibits the production of cholesterol very well. But at what price?

Sally Fallon and Mary G. Enig say all physicians know that every cell membrane in our body contains cholesterol. It makes our cells waterproof and if cholesterol levels are not high enough, the cell membrane becomes spongy, the body sees this as a problem and release hormones that moves cholesterol from one part of the body to the areas where it is lacking. Cholesterol is the body's repair substance: scar tissue contains high levels of cholesterol, including scar tissue in the arteries.

Cholesterol is the forerunner to vitamin D and the bile salts are made of cholesterol, which is required for the digestion of fat. Therefore people with low cholesterol often have trouble digesting fats. Cholesterol also functions as a powerful antioxidant, which is protecting us from cancer and aging.

Cholesterol furthermore plays a vital role in neurological functions such as memory, the uptake of hormones in the brain, including serotonin, the body's feel-good chemical.

Finally, cholesterol plays a role in regulating blood sugar levels and mineral balance as well as the production of sex hormones, including testosterone, estrogen and progesterone.

Low cholesterol can therefore lead to blood sugar problems, edema, mineral deficiencies, chronic inflammation, and difficulty in healing, allergies, asthma, reduced libido, infertility and various reproductive problems.

Did Statins Come to the Rescue?

Statin drugs replaced the cholesterol-lowering drugs which prevented the absorption from the gut. But those drugs often had immediate and unpleasant side effects, such as nausea, indigestion and constipation and most of the times it did not lower the cholesterol by any significant margins.

So statins entered the market and showed great promise when it did not cause nausea or indigestion and proved extremely effective in lowering cholesterol, often lowering cholesterol levels by 50 points or more. The statin industry was born and more than 30 million Americans are taking it.

Big success? Not really. Lately there are growing reports of serious side effects.

Muscle Pain and Weakness

The most common side effect, which involves up to 98% of users is complains about muscle pain and weakness when taking statins.

Tahoe City resident Doug Peterson developed slurred speech, balance problems and severe fatigue after three years on Lipitor-- for two and a half years, he had no side effects at all. It began with restless sleep patterns--twitching and flailing his arms. Loss of balance followed and the beginning of what Doug calls the "statin shuffle"--a slow, wobbly walk across the room. Fine motor skills suffered next. It took him five minutes to write four words, much of which was illegible. Cognitive function also declined. It was hard to convince his doctors that Lipitor could be the culprit, but when he finally stopped taking it, his coordination and memory improved.

This is in all likelihood created because of the destruction of Co-Q in the body by the statins.

John Altrocchi took Mevacor for three years without side effects; then he developed calf pain so severe he could hardly walk. He also experienced episodes of temporary memory loss.

For some, however, muscle problems show up shortly after treatment begins. Ed Ontiveros began having muscle problems within 30 days of taking Lipitor. He fell in the bathroom and had trouble getting up. The weakness subsided when he went off Lipitor. In another case, reported in the medical journal Heart, a patient developed rhabdomyolysis after a single dose of a statin.6 Heel pain from heel spurs (plantar fasciitis) is another common complaint among those taking statin drugs. One correspondent reported the onset of pain in the feet shortly after beginning statin treatment. She had visited an evangelist, requesting that he pray for her sore feet. He inquired whether she was taking Lipitor. When she said yes, he told her that his feet had also hurt when he took Lipitor.

Effects on the Nervous System

Researchers did a study of half a million people and found that people who took statins were more likely to develop polyneuropathy (weakness, tingling and pain in the hands and feet as well as difficulty walking). They found that:

- Taking statins for one year raised the risk of nerve damage by about 15%

- Taking statins for two or more years, the risk rose to 26 %

Dr. Golomb found that there is a 14-fold increased risk of developing nerve problems when using statins for two or more years.

The damage is often irreversible. People who take large doses for a long time may be left with permanent nerve damage, even after they stop taking the drug.

Heart Failure

In the United States, the number of heart attack has declined slightly but the, number of cases of heart failure cases has increased to wipe out the gains. Heart failure more than doubled from 1989 to 1997. Please note that statins were approved in 1987.

Cardiologist Peter Langsjoen studied 20 patients with completely normal heart function. After six months on a low dose of 20 mg of Lipitor a day, two-thirds of the patients had abnormalities in the heart's filling phase, when the muscle fills with blood. According to Langsjoen, this malfunction is due to Co-Q10 depletion. Without Co-Q10, the cell's mitochondria are inhibited from producing energy, leading to muscle pain and weakness. The heart is especially susceptible because it uses so much energy.

Of the nine controlled trials on statin-induced Co-Q10 depletion in humans, eight showed significant Co-Q10 depletion leading to decline in left ventricular function and biochemical imbalances.

Almost without exception, people suffering from heart failure are put on statin drugs, even if their cholesterol is already low. However a recent study actually advises the opposite – people with chronic heart failure benefit from having high levels of cholesterol rather than low.

Researchers in Hull, UK followed 114 heart failure patients for at least 12 months. Survival was 78 percent at 12 months and 56 percent at 36 months. They found that for every point of decrease in serum cholesterol, there was a 36 percent increase in the risk of death within 3 years.

Dizziness

Dizziness is commonly associated with statin use. According to Dr. Golumb, dizziness is a common adverse effect of using statins, the elderly may be particularly sensitive to drops in blood pressure.

Cognitive Impairment

Dr. Golomb has found that 15 percent of statin patients develop some cognitive side effects, some of them as serious as global transient amnesia--complete memory loss for a brief or lengthy period.

Many people report baffling incidents involving complete loss of memory--arriving at a store and not remembering why they are there, unable to remember their name or the names of their loved ones, unable to find their way home in the car.

The November 2003 issue of Smart Money describes the case of Mike Hope, owner of a successful ophthalmologic supply company: "There's an awkward silence when you ask Mike Hope his age. He doesn't change the subject or stammer, or make a silly joke about how he stopped counting at 21. He simply doesn't remember. Ten seconds pass. Then 20. Finally an answer comes to him. 'I'm 56,' he says. Close, but not quite. 'I will be 56 this year.' Later, if you happen to ask him about the book he's reading, you'll hit another roadblock. He can't recall the title, the author or the plot." Statin use since 1998 has caused his speech and memory to fade. He was forced to close his business and went on Social Security 10 years early. Things improved when he discontinued Lipitor in 2002, but he is far from complete recovery--he still cannot sustain a conversation. What Lipitor did was turn Mike Hope into an old man when he was in the prime of life.

The pharmaceutical industry strongly denies that statins can cause amnesia but in several statin trials memory loss has shown up as one of the side effects.

An article in Pharmacotherapy, December 2003, for example, reports two cases of cognitive impairment associated with Lipitor and Zocor. Both patients suffered progressive cognitive decline that reversed completely within a month after discontinuation of the statins. A study conducted at the University of Pittsburgh showed that patients treated with statins for six months compared poorly with patients on a placebo in solving complex mazes, psychomotor skills and memory tests.

Cancer

In every study with rodents to date, without exception, statins have caused cancer. The question is why have we not seen such a dramatic correlation in human studies? The answer is that it takes longer to develop cancer in the human body and most statin trials do not go on longer than two or three years.

However in the CARE trial it was shown that breast cancer rates of those taking a statin went up 1,500%

Even the manufacturers of statins have admitted that statins lower the immune system, an effect that can lead to cancer and infectious disease.

And now for the crazy part:

Because of the effect of lowering the immune system; they are now recommending that statins should be used for inflammatory arthritis and as an immune suppressor for transplant patients!

Pancreatic Rot

There are several reports of pancreatitis (infection/inflammation of the pancreas) in patients taking statins.

One paper describes the case of a 49-year-old woman who was admitted to the hospital with diarrhea and septic shock one month after beginning treatment with lovastatin. She died after prolonged hospitalization; the cause of death was necrotizing pancreatitis. Her doctors noted that the patient had no evidence of common risk factors for acute pancreatitis, such as biliary tract disease or alcohol use. "Prescribers of statins (particularly simvastatin and lovastatin) should take into account the possibility of acute pancreatitis in patients who develop abdominal pain within the first weeks of treatment with these drugs," they warned.

Depression

Numerous studies have linked low cholesterol with depression.

One of the most recent found that women with low cholesterol are twice as likely to suffer from depression and anxiety. Researchers from Duke University Medical Center carried out personality trait measurements on 121 young women aged 18 to 27. They found that 39 percent of the women with low cholesterol levels scored

high on personality traits that signaled proneness to depression,
compared to 19 percent of women with normal or high levels of
cholesterol. In addition, one in three of the women with low
cholesterol levels scored high on anxiety indicators, compared to
21 percent with normal levels.

Yet the author of the study, Dr. Edward Suarez, cautioned women
with low cholesterol against eating "foods such as cream cakes" to
raise cholesterol, warning that these types of food "can cause
heart disease." In previous studies on men, Dr. Suarez found that
men who lower their cholesterol levels with medication have
increased rates of suicide and violent death, leading the
researchers to theorize "that low cholesterol levels were causing
mood disturbances."

So Are There Any Benefits?

Most doctors are convinced and try to convince their patients that
the benefits of statin drugs far outweigh the side effects. They
have all the statistics to show that statin use has lowered the
number of coronary deaths.

However Dr. Ravnskov has pointed out in his book The Cholesterol
Myths, the results of the major studies up to the year 2000--the
4S, WOSCOPS, CARE, AFCAPS and LIPID studies--generally showed

only small differences and these differences were often statistically insignificant and independent of the amount of cholesterol lowering achieved. In two studies, EXCEL, and FACAPT/TexCAPS, more deaths occurred in the treatment group compared to controls. Dr. Ravnskov's 1992 meta-analysis of 26 controlled cholesterol-lowering trials found an equal number of cardiovascular deaths in the treatment and control groups and a greater number of total deaths in the treatment groups. An analysis of all the big controlled trials reported before 2000 found that long-term use of statins for primary prevention of heart disase produced a 1 percent greater risk of death over 10 years compared to a placebo.

Even more recently studies fail to provide any more justification for the current campaign to put as many people as possible on statin drugs.

Please Read the Rest

I would like to encourage you to read the full article by these two brilliant scientists on the website below. They also quote the details of a long list of case studies to prove their point which is well worth the read.
www.westonaprice.org/moderndiseases/statin.html

Finally the Costs

Statin drugs are very expensive, costing between $900 and $1400 per year per patient. Statins are the most widely sold pharmaceutical drug, making up 6.5% of market share and $12.5 billion dollars in revenue for the industry.

According to the National Health Service in the UK doctors wrote 31 million prescriptions for statins in 2003, up from 1 million in 1995 at a cost of 7 billion pounds and that's just in one tiny island. In the US, statins currently bring in $12.5 billion annually for the pharmaceutical industry. Sales of Lipitor, the number-one-selling statin, were projected to hit $10 billion in 2005.

In the WOSCOP clinical trial, healthy people with high cholesterol were treated with statins, the five-year death rate for treated subjects was reduced by a mere 0.6 %.

As Dr. Ravnskov points out, to achieve that slight reduction about 165 healthy people had to be treated for five years to extend one life by five years. The cost for that one life comes to $1.2 million dollars.

After reading this full article by Sally Fallon and Mary G. Enig on this website and many other cases I could not help but think: "When is someone going to take them to court?

Aspirin and Nonsteroidal Anti-inflammatory Drugs (NSAIDs)

Many of the conventional medical practitioners prescribe an aspirin a day for their patients. They believe that it acts as a blood thinner and that it will prevent clogging of the arteries because the blood is thinner. However it has been proven to be a flawed theory - the benefits does not come because of the thinning of the blood but because it actually helps to prevent and or fight inflammation.

It has been shown that continued use of anti-inflammatory drugs like aspirin, disprin or other nonsteroidal, anti-inflammatory drugs can help to prevent heart attack and strokes can increase the survival rate but there are a few side effects to consider.

Taking aspirin and/or any other (NSAIDs) daily can have serious side effects that need to be considered before using it, says **Dr. Gordon.** *"These can cause internal bleeding, plus liver and kidney damage, and are linked to 20,000 deaths and over 125,000 hospitalizations annually. Fortunately, we do not have to rely on such drugs, nor wait for new drugs to be developed, for there are a number of safe, natural substances that can be used instead, which are documented to have the same health benefits without the side effects."*

Angioplasty and Bypass Surgery

Angioplasty and bypass surgery is not justified and in fact is aggravating the very condition it is supposed to treat.

More than 15 years ago (1992), Nortin Hadler, M.D., Professor of Medicine at the University of North Carolina School of Medicine, wrote:

- Not one single one of the 250,000 balloon angioplasties performed in 1991 can be justified.

- Only 3% to 5% of the 300,000 coronary bypass surgeries done in 1991 were actually required.

About 10 years earlier at a symposium of the American Heart Association by Henry Mcintosh, M.D., said that bypass surgery should be limited to patients with crippling angina who do not respond to more conservative treatment.

It has been proven beyond doubt that most angioplasty and bypass surgery do not extend life after a heart attack.

In a 1997 report in the **New England Journal of Medicine**, it was stated that:

- *The death rate of U.S. and Canadian heart attack patients after one year was 34%.*

- *Among the U.S. patients, 12% had received angioplasty and 11% had bypass surgery, compared to the Canadian patients, with only 1 .5% receiving angioplasty and only 1.4% had bypass surgery.*

- *U.S. patients are also five times more likely (34.9% to 6.7%) to have coronary angiography (catheterization of heart arteries) than Canadians, with one-year survival rates between patients in both countries basically remaining equal.*

Apart from the trauma and scarring of these procedures some other serious side effects were also prevalent. Researchers found that 5 years after heart bypass surgery, 42% of patients *"show a significant decline on tests of mental ability, probably from brain damage caused by the surgery."* The researchers also noted that: *"it highlights an ugly truth that surgeons know but are not eager to discuss with patients."*

Furthermore researchers also found that bypass surgery after a heart attack or angina may actually increase the risk of stroke within months after the procedure is performed.

Heart Catheterization

This is a test where they insert a catheter (tube) through the neck to measure blood pressure inside the heart. But this procedure has never undergone strict scientific trials and remains experimental. A study in 1996 study concluded that this procedure can significantly increase a patient's risk of death.

In spite of this, more than 500,000 patients in the U.S. receive heart catheterization annually.

According to Dr Julian Whitaker, M.D., author of Reversing Heart Disease, catheterization *"leads to a dramatic increase in the use of bypass surgery and angioplasty because physicians then try to open up observed blockages."* But research shows that when catheterization is followed by either of these procedures, the death rate of heart attack survivors increases by 36%!

Alternative Treatment - Overview

Let us have a look at the alternative treatment options that can prevent, cure and reverse heart disease.

Alternative Health Practitioners are saying:

"Although heart disease causes half of all deaths in the United States it is one of the most preventable chronic degenerative diseases. ... The risk of heart attacks and strokes can be greatly decreased through dietary changes, exercise, stress reduction, and nutritional supplementation, as well as other alternative therapies".

Natural treatments provide a wide range of extremely effective and less risky options to prevent and reduce the risk of heart disease. These same treatments will also be beneficial to those already suffering from heart disease and has proved in numerous cases to reverse heart disease.

These treatments include dietary changes, nutritional supplementation, herbal medicine, alternative treatments such as chelation therapy, detoxification, oxygen therapy, exercise and stress reduction, traditional Chinese medicine, and Ayurvedic medicine.

Although initial damage done to the arteries can cause the buildup of plaque, it can be corrected and reversed through diet and nutritional supplements.

In order to prevent heart disease it is of the utmost importance to:

- Stop/prevent the oxidation of LDL cholesterol

- Lower the level of LDL cholesterol because then there is less to oxidize.

- Increase the level of HDL (high density lipoprotein) cholesterol, which transports the LDL away from your arteries and back to your liver.

There are a variety of supplements and herbs that will help lower LDL and raise HDL or both at the same time and also help prevent the oxidation of LDL cholesterol.

A few facts to remember:

- 85% percent of all heart disease is caused by vulnerable plaque.

- Conventional cardiovascular diagnostic tests cannot detect vulnerable plaque.

- MRI scanning and darkfield microscopy are much * Vulnerable plaque is usually triggered by chronic infection and people at risk of heart disease should be screened for infectious agents, as well as oxidized cholesterol, fibrinogen and homocysteine levels, and free-radical damage.

Below is a quick summary of what will be covered in the rest of this book.

In your diet:

- Eat organic foods (free of pesticides, herbicides, steroids, and antibiotics) whenever possible.

- Increase fiber from green leafy vegetables, complex carbohydrates, fresh raw fruits, bran, whole grains, and psyllium.

- Use monounsaturated oils (like olive oil), omega-3 oils (fish oils or flaxseed oil), and omega-6 oils (borage oil or evening primrose oil).

- Avoid processed foods (with additives and preservatives or foods containing powdered eggs or powdered milk) and irradiated foods whenever possible.

- Reduce intake of harmful fats, especially fried foods, animal fats, and partially hydrogenated oils, and eliminate sugar and tobacco.

Take Supplements:

- Introduce a proper nutritional supplementation program into your diet. It has been shown that it can significantly improve cardiovascular conditions, as well as prevent them from occurring in the first place.

- Useful nutrients include beta carotene; vitamins B3 (niacin), B6, B12, C, and E; folic acid; the minerals calcium, chromium, magnesium, potassium, and selenium; the amino acids L-arginine, L-taurine, and L-carnitine; coenzyme Q10 and pycnogenol.

Use Herbs:

- Useful herbs for heart disease include foxglove (Thgitalis purpurea), hawthorn berry, garlic, ginger,

- Both exercise and stress reduction can help mitigate heart disease risk and improve recovery.

There are Other Treatment Options

There are other treatment options which have proved to be much more effective with less side effects and dangers than conventional treatments such as angioplasty, bypass surgery and cholesterol lowering drugs.

- Chelation Therapy

- Enzyme Therapy

- Oxygen Therapy

These therapies will be discussed in much more detail later in the book.

Alternative Treatment - Diet

Dietary measures have proved to be highly effective in reversing heart disease.

Dean Ornish, M.D.,Assistant Clinical Professor of Medicine at the University of California in San Francisco, developed a regimen using a strict vegetarian diet combined with exercise and stress reduction which he calls the "reversal diet". It is almost entirely free of cholesterol, animal fats, and oils and proved that his patients who follow this diet improved dramatically over those who followed a diet high in fat.

Dr. Cowden, however, says that it is not the low level of cholesterol Dr. Ornish's diet which is beneficial, but that the success should rather be ascribed to the fact that it contains low levels of methioninc (an amino acid found in red meat, milk, and milk products, and a precursor to homocysteine, a free radical capable of oxidizing cholesterol) and to a high intake of vegetables and grains. These foods are rich in those vitamins (B6, C, and E, and beta carotene) that act as co-factors for antioxidants and antiatherogenics (substances preventing atherosclerosis).

Cut down on the intake of red meat, milk and milk products and increase the intake of vegetables.

Dr. Passwater suggests, to reduce oxidized cholesterol in the bloodstream, a diet with less than 30% of daily calories from fat combined with a nutritional supplementation program. He says: "What needs to be done is to first control the LDL cholesterol through diet, then raise the antioxidant level to prevent oxidized cholesterol from doing damage."

A healthy diet will limit food, such as red meat and fried foods containing oxidized or hydrogenated fats that generates homocysteine and will include supplements that fight oxidation (antioxidants).

Onions, apples and green or black tea can also contribute to a healthy heart. These items contain high levels of bioflavonoid and quercetin with very effective antioxidant properties. Bioflavonoids enhance the good activities of vitamin C and help to keep the immune system strong. A study has shown that people with high levels of quercetin had a 53% lower risk of heart disease than those with the lowest levels.

Furthermore, apples, dark chocolate and green or black tea are also rich in catechins, another beneficial bioflavonoid.

In the Netherlands during a 10 year study it was found that people who consumed an average of 72 mg of catechins per day, which can be obtained from 4 apples, 2 cups of tea, or a small piece of chocolate daily were 51% less likely to die of ischemic heart disease compared to those who consumed the least amount. Ischemic heart disease is caused by clogged arteries, which reduce the amount of blood and oxygen supply to the heart.

Eat apples every day, replace coffee (both caffeinated and de caffeinated) with tea (black or green) also eat a small piece of dark chocolate every day.

Good Fats and Bad Fats

At this stage it is probably important to understand that not all fats (oils) are created equal. Our bodies need fats because it helps with absorption of nutrients from our food, nerve transmission, maintenance of the cell membranes and many other vital functions.

Bad fats contribute to weight gain, inflammation, heart disease and cancer while good fats promote a healthy body. It is therefore important to replace the bad fats with good fats in our diet.

The Good Fats

The good fats consist of 2 groups, Monounsaturated Fats and Polyunsaturated Fats.

Monounsaturated Fats

Monounsaturated fats are those fats that we find in most nuts; peanuts, almonds, walnuts and pistachios. We also encounter it in avocado, canola and olive oil. It has been proven that monounsaturated fats help in weight loss, lowering of total cholesterol and LDL cholesterol while increasing HDL cholesterol.

Polyunsaturated Fats

Polyunsaturated fats are encountered in seafood like salmon and fish oil. It has also been proven that Polyunsaturated fats lower total cholesterol and LDL cholesterol while it raises HDL cholesterol.

The Bad Fats

The bad fats consist of 2 groups, Saturated Fats and Trans Fats.

Saturated Fats

Saturated fats are encountered in red meat, dairy, fatty beef, lamb, pork, poultry with skin, beef fat (tallow), lard and cream, butter, cheese and other dairy products made from whole or reduced-fat (2 percent) milk, eggs and seafood as well as some plant oils such as coconut oil, palm oil and palm kernel oil. It has been shown to raise total blood cholesterol as well as LDL cholesterol.

Saturated fats and trans fats (from hydrogenated oils) create a serious risk for heart disease. In a study that tracked the medical conditions of 5,200 men (age 42-53) over a period of 22 years the finding was:

The men with higher blood levels of Saturated fats and trans fats were up to 70% more likely to experience sudden death form heart disease than the men with lower levels.

Trans Fats

Trans fats are the real bad brother of the two. Certain oils are "hydrogenated" (hydrogen is added) in order to have a longer shelf life and are found in many of the commercially packaged foods, fried food such as French fries in fast food chains, packaged snacks such as microwaved popcorn as well as in vegetable shortening and margarine. Eating these types of foods poses a serious risk to our health as you will see below.

It is a well-known fact that saturated and trans fats increase the levels of LDL and therefore increase the risk of heart disease. More recently it was found that trans fats are actually much worse than saturated fats.

29 healthy, non-smoking people were divided into 2 groups to follow a diet high in trans fats (9.2% of total calories) for one group and the other group on a diet with the same amount of saturated fats. The findings were:

That the trans-fat diet reduced blood vessel function by 29% and also reduced healthy HDL levels by 20%, compared to the saturated-fat diet.

Omega Fatty Acids

These days there are also a lot of talk and hype about omega fatty acids and the words like Omega 3, Omega 6 and Omega 9 are being thrown around every day.

What are Omega Fatty Acids?

Omega fatty acids are also called essential fatty acids. Essential because the body cannot produce Omega fatty acids and you have to provide it to your body through your diet. But note that only Omega 3 and 6 are essential not Omega 9 because our body can actually manufacture it. The omega fatty acids are vital for your body functions in order to maintain cellular health, prevent inflammation, maintain the nervous system and fight certain illnesses.

Many studies have shown that Omega fatty acids can prevent cancer, help with mental health disorders, lower LDL cholesterol, raise HDL cholesterol and many other benefits.

There are three different kinds of Omega fatty acids; Omega 3, 6, and 9. Each of them has a different chemical structure therefore the different numbers 3, 6 and 9.

Omega 3

Omega 3 fatty acids are in oily fishes and in fish oil supplements. Omega 3s have been shown to help prevent and cure heart disease (see studies below), lower high blood pressure, fight inflammation, assist those with arthritis and other autoimmune disorders and help with mental disorders and improve people with ADD and ADHD as well.

Omega-3 fatty acids are the most important of the three fatty acids. The most important reason for this is because they suppress inflammation, which is the cause of many of the degenerative diseases, including heart disease.

In order to lower the level of homocysteine it is of vital importance that you complement your diet with essential fatty acids (EFAs) which is found in the Omega-3 oils from flaxseed oil, ocean algae or from cold saltwater fish, such as Scandinavian salmon, orange roughy, halibut and other types of fish and seafood. These oils are extremely useful in reducing LDL cholesterol and have proved to prevent heart attacks by eliminating clotting and arterial damage.

<u>Omega 6</u>

Omega 6 fatty acids are in plant sources like nuts and flax seeds. These essential fatty acids have many of the same benefits as Omega 3. It has been shown to reduce inflammation and help people with arthritis and other autoimmune diseases, have very positive effects on the skin diseases such as acne and psoriasis. It is also very helpful in the prevention and treatment of heart disease (see studies below).

It is very important that we try to balance the ratio of intake of Omega 3 to Omega 6. Most of us get too much Omega 6 in our diets. Omega 6 can be found plentifully in many vegetable cooking oils such as soybean oil, sunflower oil, canola oil and corn oil (but not olive oil). They're also common ingredients in many of the foods we consume, which is why most of us have a heavily imbalanced ratio of Omega-6's to 3's.

Omega 6 prevents the stickiness of blood platelets, allowing blood to pass through the arteries without danger of clotting. The best sources of Omega 6 are borage oil, black currant oil, and evening primrose oil and grapeseed oil which contain 76% linoleic acid (an omega-6 oil). Grapeseed oil has a high concentration of vitamin E a vital antioxidant.

<u>Omega 9</u>

This is the lesser-known fatty acid of the three. However Omega 9 does play a large role in a healthy body. On the other hand it is the most abundant fatty acids of all in nature and are not in short supply in our diets. They are also not considered essential because our bodies can make Omega-9 from unsaturated fat.

The best source of Omega 9 is olive oil. Olive oil has been shown to be an extremely effective preventer of disease but this is mainly due to the high polyphenol content rather than to its fatty acid content.

Olive oil should be used for all cooking because of its strong antioxidant, anti-inflammatory, anti-clotting and antibacterial effects.

Omega 9 is also found in animal fat other vegetable oils and avocados and does play a vital role in cancer prevention and heart protection; however these should generally make up a smaller part of your diet because they can include saturated fats, which are harmful to the heart in larger quantities.

Getting More Essential Fatty Acids in Your Diet

The best sources of essential fatty acids are – fish, flaxseed, avocados, olive oil, grapeseed oil, nuts etc.

You should make sure that you have healthy servings of those in order to maintain a healthy body and heart.

Things have been made much easier with the availability of all the Omega fatty acids in supplement forms. These supplements are usually in a capsule form and are easy to take, easy to digest and easy to remember.

Foods for Cholesterol Control

There are many different types of foods that can assist you in the fight to lower LDL cholesterol and improve HDL cholesterol. Below are the ones that are most recommended by alternative health practitioners.

Oat Bran: Can Lower Cholesterol by 10%

Amy Rothenberg, N.D., a naturopathic physician in Enfield, Connecticut, says *"Oat bran is rich in soluble fiber, a substance that binds with cholesterol in the intestine and ushers it out of the body. Eating 3/4 cup of cooked oat bran cereal a day can lower cholesterol by 10%. However, if you're more likely to eat an oat bran muffin, that works, too."*

Onions and Garlic: Don't Mind the Smell

Mark Stengler, N.D., a naturopathic physician in San Diego says: *"Cook with garlic and onions whenever possible. Both have been shown to cut cholesterol. Or you can take garlic supplements, following the dosage recommendations on the label".*

In the chapter about herbs I will give you much more information about the proven benefits of garlic.

Walnuts: Be a Health Nut

Kitty Gurkin Rosati, R.D., a registered dietitian and nutrition director of the Rice Diet Program at Duke University in Durham, North Carolina says: *"Walnuts contain alpha-linolenic acid, which can help lower cholesterol. Other good sources of this good-for-you fat include olive oil, flaxseed oil, linseed oil, canola oil, soybean oil, and purslane, a salad green. To get a double dose, sauté purslane in a teaspoon of olive oil"*

Lecithin: Dissolves Cholesterol

Dr. Rothenberg says:*"Lecithin granules contain phosphatidylcholine, which helps liquefy cholesterol in your body so it doesn't end up frozen in arterial plaques".*

It is recommended that you get at least 1 tablespoon of granules in per day; sprinkle it on your oat bran or mix it into a healthy smoothie

Soy: Any Form Will Do

Dr Strengler says: *"Tofu, tempeh, and other soy foods contain compounds called isoflavones which can help lower cholesterol. An easy way to incorporate isoflavones into your diet is to add soy protein powder to a shake. Or eat more tofu and miso, two popular soy foods that are versatile and easy to cook with".*

Apple-Cider Vinegar – Melts Away Arterial Plaque

Dr. Patrick Quillin, R.D. Ph.D. director of the Rational Healing Institute in Tulsa, Oklahoma says that apple-cider vinegar enhances the friendly bacteria in the body which helps to reduce cholesterol and immune functions. He recommends that you take

1 teaspoon 3 times a day on salads or mixed with regular apple cider.

The Encyclopaedia of Natural Medicine Recommends

In their book Encyclopedia of Natural Medicine Revised 2nd Edition: Michael Murray N.D. and Joseph Pizzorno N.D. recommends the following approach to lower cholesterol.

The most important approach to lowering a high cholesterol level is a healthful diet and lifestyle.

The dietary guidelines are straightforward:

- *Eat less saturated fat and cholesterol by reducing or eliminating the amount of animal products in the diet*

- *Eat more fiber-rich plant foods (fruits, vegetables, grains, and legumes).*

- *Lose weight if necessary*

The lifestyle guidelines are:

- *Get regular aerobic exercise.*

- *Don't smoke.*

- *Reduce or eliminate consumption of coffee (caffeine and decaffeinated)*

In many cases, diet alone is not enough to get cholesterol levels into the preferred ranges. However, there are several natural supplements and compounds that can lower cholesterol levels and significantly reduce risk factors for heart disease.

The natural alternatives offer significant advantages over standard drug therapy. See the next chapter for natural supplements.

Michael Murray and Joseph Pizzorno also suggest that we make the following practical changes to our daily diets:

- Cut out Red meat and eat more Fish and white meat or poultry.

- Cut out Hamburgers and hot dogs and eat more Soy-based alternatives.

- Cut out Eggs and eat more Egg Beaters and similar products and tofu.

- Cut out High-fat dairy products and eat more Low-fat or nonfat dairy products.

- Cut out Butter, lard, and other saturated fats and eat more olive oil.

- Cut out Ice cream, pie, coke, cookies, etc. and eat more fruits.

- Cut out Refined cereals, white bread, etc. and eat more Whole grains, whole wheat bread.

- Cut out Fried foods, fatty snack foods and eat more Vegetables and fresh salads.

- Cut out Salt and salty foods and eat more Low sodium, light salt.

- Cut out Coffee and soft drinks and eat more Herbal teas, fresh fruit and vegetable juices.

Eat to Prevent Heart Disease

Cardiologist Dr. Cowden, provides the following dietary guidelines to prevent heart disease:

- Eat minimally processed foods (avoid additives and preservatives or foods containing powdered eggs or powdered milk).

- Buy organic foods (free of pesticides, herbicides, steroids, and antibiotics) whenever possible, especially when buying meats and dairy products.

- Avoid irradiated foods whenever possible.

- Increase fiber from green leafy vegetables, fresh raw fruits, bran, whole grains, and psyllium.

- Reduce fat intake, especially fried foods, animal fats, and partially hydrogenated oils. Increase complex carbohydrates such as whole grains, beans, seeds, and potatoes.

- Use monounsaturated oils (such as cold-pressed olive oil), omega-3 oils (linseed/flaxseed oil or oils from deep ocean fish), and omega-6 oils (borage, black currant oil, or evening primrose oil).

- Reduce meat, sugar, tobacco, and alcohol consumption, which are all sources of free radicals.

Dr. Cowden puts many of his heart patients through a detoxification process consisting of a vegetarian diet, vegetable juices mixed with garlic and (in some cases) cayenne, as well as low-temperature saunas. His program assists to clean the body of harmful toxins which damage the artery walls and buildup arterial plaque.

The Anti-Inflammation Diet

Jack Challem's book the "The Inflammation Syndrome" is devoted to the treatment and prevention of inflammation in the body which is causing a myriad of diseases including heart disease.

I would like to recommend that you get yourself a copy of this book and study it. You can order it from here www.stopinflammation.com

Please note: *I don't know the author, have never met him and are not getting any benefits whatsoever from promoting his book or website. I am recommending his book purely because I think it is most probably the best resource (for lay people) on the topic of inflammation available.*

Many of the leading health organisations like the Arthritis Foundation and the American College of Rheumatology have for decades been denying that diet can cure arthritis and/or inflammation. In fact they have been describing it as quackery.

On the other hand, alternative health practitioners have for almost 100 years been saying that diet could and in fact do fight inflammation. In recent times the conventional health practitioners are being overwhelmed with evidence to substantiate this fact.

Researchers have amassed data from 1911 showing that diet programs could and in fact do produce remission of inflammatory reactions in the body.

It has been found that certain foods contain allergens that irritate the body which the body have to constantly fight and adapt to. Some of these allergens occur naturally in certain foods while others occur in the food additives. Some of the most commonly known foods that cause inflammation are wheat, corn, milk, and dairy products, and red meat. Common allergens like casein (in dairy products) and gluten (in grains) are quick to spark the inflammatory cascade.

In addition, it has also been proven that the nightshade family of foods also contains these allergens and it is better to avoid them as much as you can in your diet. Nightshade foods include; Potatoes, Tomatoes, Eggplant (Aubergine), Bell peppers (green, red, yellow, cherry), Hot peppers (long & red, red cluster), Chili peppers, (basically all peppers, except, white and black pepper), Paprika, Tabasco, Belladonna (used in homeopathy) Cayenne pepper (capsicum) Pimento, Henbane, Mandrake, Jimson weed and Tobacco. Yes tobacco is a nightshade!

Allergic reactions can occur to one or many of the above. For people who are outright allergic to nightshade foods common symptoms are nausea, diarrhoea, dizziness, and inflammation, stiffness in the joints, migraines and weakness/fatigue. Furthermore, lowering the fat intake in your diet significantly lowers the inflammation in your body and it is recommended that the elimination of animal and vegetable fats may be helpful.

As mentioned before, the Omega-3 oils found in flaxseed oil and in cold-water fish, such as tuna, salmon, herring, trout, mackerel, sardines, and cod liver, are excellent inflammation fighters. So is GLA (gamma-linolenic acid), an omega-6 oil that is present in primrose oil, borage oil, and black currant seed oil.

It was also found that people who follow a more "primitive" diet (in other words avoiding refined foods and food additives) than those who don't, have a much lower incidence of inflammatory diseases such as rheumatoid arthritis, heart disease etc.

Therefore, it is highly recommended that you limit or eliminate sugar, saturated fat, meats, and refined carbohydrates from your diet and to eat copious amounts of cooked vegetables, olive oil, fresh fruits, whole grains and unrefined carbohydrates. Here are the foods to avoid and the foods to eat:

Foods to Avoid:

- Avoid Sugar

- Artificial sweeteners

- Processed foods

- Junk food

- Red meat

- Pork

- White bread and pasta

- Frozen and canned foods

Foods to Eat:

- Wild Salmon and other fish

- Nuts and Seeds- walnuts, flax and pumpkin

- Olive Oil and Canola Oil

- Soy

- Fruits- especially strawberries & blueberries

- Vegetables - especially leafy greens

- Oats and other whole grains

- Water

Always remember that olive oil is rich in vitamin E, a courageous and extremely efficient soldier in the war against inflammation. Olive oil also contains polyphenolic compounds that have been shown to have both anti-inflammatory and antioxidative effects. So, consuming olive oil instead of those other pro-inflammatory fats and vegetable oils will significantly reduce the inflammatory processes.

You should eat at least five or more servings of fruits and vegetables each day. Green vegetables and whole fruits are very important sources of dietary fibre. The pigments in brightly coloured fruits, vegetables and berries contain many phytochemicals that have anti-inflammatory properties. For instance quercetin in apples and red onion skins has strong anti-inflammatory properties.

By now you know that if you eat anti-inflammatory foods regularly you can and will reduce inflammation in the body. Below is a list of anti-inflammatory and other healthy foods to help you create a healthy diet and bring a balance to inflammation in your body. Please take note that this is not a comprehensive list. I included it into this book as a starting point just to demonstrate to you the many food choices we have that are much healthier than the ones we sometimes choose.

Oils

Choose: All cooking should be done with Extra Virgin Olive Oil and/or Grapeseed oil and/or Canola Oil. Use Avocado Oil or Olive Oil for salad dressings.

Avoid: Sunflower, Safflower, Peanut Oil, Butter, Lard , Gravy , Cream sauce , Non-dairy creamers , Hydrogenated Margarine and Shortening , Cocoa butter, Coconut, Palm and Palm-kernel oils and any other oils except those mentioned above.

Vegetables

Choose: Green leafy vegetables, green and brightly colored vegetables, Bok Choy, Broccoli, Broccoli Sprouts, Brussels Sprouts, Cabbage, Carrots, Cauliflower, Chard, Collards, Fennel Bulb, Garlic, Green Beans, Green Onions/Spring Onions, Kale. Leeks, Olives, Spinach, Sweet potatoes Turnip Greens

Avoid: Nightshade vegetables like Potatoes, Tomatoes, Eggplant (Aubergine), Bell Peppers (green, red, yellow, cherry), Hot Peppers (long & red, red cluster), Chili Peppers, (basically all peppers, except, white and black pepper), Paprika, Tabasco,

Belladonna (used in homeopathy) Cayenne pepper (capsicum) Pimento, Henbane, Mandrake, Jimson Weed and Tobacco. Also avoid Coconut, Creamy sauces, Fried or Breaded Vegetables

Fruits

Choose: Acerola (West Indian), Cherries, Apples, Avocados, Black Currants, Blueberries, Fresh Pineapple, Guavas, Kiwifruit, Kumquats, Mulberries, Papaya, Raspberries, Rhubarb, Strawberries. Most berries are packed with anti-inflammatory phytochemicals and anti-oxidants.

Avoid: Canned fruit packed in heavy syrup

Protein

Choose: Cold water oily fish, Cod, Halibut, Herring, Oysters, Rainbow Trout, Salmon, Sardines, Snapper Fish, Striped Bass, Tuna, Whitefish, Skinless white-meat Poultry, Nuts, Eggs, Legumes and Seeds. When you do eat red meat, choose lean cuts of Bison, Venison and other Game Meats, or the lowest-fat cuts of Beef, preferably grass-fed beef. Soybeans, Tofu, and Soy milk are three great sources of proteins that may help to reduce your inflammation.

Avoid: Milk and Dairy Products, Organ meats, such as liver, Fatty and Marbled Meats, Spareribs, Processed meats such as Cold cuts, Frankfurters, Hot Dogs, Bacon, Fried Breaded or Canned Meats.

Carbohydrates and Fibre

Choose: Most of your carbohydrates should come from whole grains, vegetables and fruits. Whole grain products have lots of fibre which is an excellent inflammation fighter. Choose Whole-wheat flour, Whole-grain Bread (must be 100 percent whole-wheat or 100 percent whole-grain), High-Fibre Cereal, Brown Rice, Whole-Grain Pasta and Oatmeal

Avoid: Muffins (except bran), Waffles, Corn bread, Doughnuts, Biscuits, Quick breads, Granola bars, Cakes, Pies, Egg noodles, Buttered popcorn, High-fat Snack Crackers and Chips.

Nuts & Seeds

Choose: Almonds, Flaxseed/Linseed, Hazelnuts, Sunflower Seeds (But never sunflower oil for cooking!), Walnuts and Pumpkin Seeds.

Herbs & Spices

Basil, Cinnamon, Cloves, Cocoa (at least 70% cocoa chocolate), Liquorice, Mint, Oregano, Parsley, Rosemary, Thyme, Turmeric.

Drinks

Your body needs water in the form of foods and beverages every day. Other good fluid sources include 100% fruit juices (with no preservatives), herbal teas (especially green tea) and vegetable juices.

22 "Super Foods" to help Prevent and Cure Heart Disease

Below is a list of 22 "super foods" to protect you from heart disease. Make sure you incorporate this into your diet.

- **Salmon** – contains large amounts of Omega-3

- **Flaxseed** (freshly ground) – contains Omega-3 fatty acids; fiber, phytoestrogens.

- **Oatmeal** - Omega-3 fatty acids; magnesium; potassium; folate; niacin; calcium; soluble fiber.

- **Black or Kidney Beans** – contains B-complex vitamins; niacin; folate; magnesium; omega-3 fatty acids; calcium; soluble fiber.

- **Almonds** – Contains plant omega-3 fatty acids; vitamin E; magnesium; fiber; heart-favorable mono- and polyunsaturated fats; phytosterols.

- **Walnuts** – Contains plant omega-3 fatty acids; vitamin E; magnesium; folate; fiber; heart-favorable mono- and polyunsaturated fats; phytosterols.

- **Red wine** – Contains catechins and reservatrol (flavonoids) improve HDL cholesterol levels.

- **Tuna** - Contains Omega-3 fatty acids; folate; niacin.

- **Tofu** - Contains Niacin; folate; calcium; magnesium; potassium.

- **Brown rice** - Contains B-complex vitamins; fiber; niacin; magnesium, fiber.

- **Soy milk** - Contains Isoflavones (a flavonoid); B-complex vitamins; niacin; folate, calcium; magnesium; potassium; phytoestrogens.

- **Blueberries** - Contains Beta-carotene and lutein (carotenoids); anthocyanin (a flavonoid); ellagic acid (a polyphenol); vitamin C; folate; calcium, magnesium; potassium; fiber. Cranberries, strawberries, raspberries are very good as well.

- **Carrots** – Contains Alpha-carotene (a carotenoid); fiber.

- **Spinach** – Contains Lutein (a carotenoid); B-complex vitamins; folate; magnesium; potassium; calcium; fiber.

- **Broccoli** – Contains Beta-carotene (a carotenoid); Vitamins C and E; potassium; folate; calcium; fiber.

- **Sweet potato** – Contains Beta-carotene (a carotenoid); vitamins A, C, E; fiber.

- **Asparagus** - Contains Beta-carotene and lutein (carotenoids); B-complex vitamins; folate; fiber.

- **Oranges** - Contains Beta-cryptoxanthin, beta- and alpha-carotene, lutein (carotenoids) and flavones (flavonoids); vitamin C; potassium; folate; fiber.

- **Acorn squash** - Contains Beta-carotene and lutein (carotenoids); B-complex and C vitamins; folate; calcium; magnesium; potassium; fiber.

- **Cantaloupe** – Contains Alpha- and beta-carotene and lutein (carotenoids); B-complex and C vitamins; folate; potassium; fiber.

- **Papaya** – Contains Beta-carotene, beta-cryptoxanthin, lutein (carotenoids); Vitamins C and E; folate; calcium; magnesium; potassium.

- **Dark chocolate** (70% or higher cocoa content - Contains resveratrol and cocoa phenols (flavonoids).

- **Tea** – Contains Catechins and flavonols (flavonoids).

Alternative Treatment – Vitamins & Minerals

Let us have a look at natural supplements and why they are achieving much, much better results than the conventional treatments such as statins and surgery.

Before I go into that, just a word of warning, many people believe they can take only supplements and that would fix the problem and they can carry on to eat and live the "good life". That is a serious mistake. Alternative treatment follows a combination of methods, diet, supplements and lifestyle. It is important to address all three factors of that combination to achieve success.

A daily regimen of supplements complimented by a healthy diet and lifestyle is an extremely efficient way of preventing heart disease. But it is important to note that supplement quantities required vary between people depending on body weight and absorption. Therefore it is critical that you consult with a nutritionally skilled physician or naturopathic physician before embarking on a routine of supplements.

Dr Matthias Rath, M.D., author of Eradicating Heart Disease, and former Director of the Linus Pauling Institute of Science and Medicine, in Palo Alto, California, is a leading advocate of nutritional supplementation to prevent and reverse heart disease. *"I firmly believe that America's number one killer can be prevented by an optimum intake of essential nutrients,"*

Dr. Rath reports one of his successes stories as follows:

A man in his fifties, who came to him after experiencing sudden cardiac failure, a severe heart muscle weakness that results in decreased pumping function and enlargement of the heart chambers.

The man was no longer able to work full-time and had to give up most physical activities. Sometimes he felt so weak he had to hold an object with both hands to keep from dropping it, and he was unable to climb stairs. Dr Rath put him on a supplement program for heart health.

"Soon, he could again fulfill his professional obligations on a regular basis and was able to undertake daily bicycle rides," Dr. *Rath says.*

After two months on the supplement program, his cardiologist found that his heart enlargement had decreased. One month later, he went on an overseas business trip and reported that physical limitations were no longer interfering with his work.

Vitamin C: The First Defense

Nobel laureate Dr Linus Pauling, Ph.D. and Dr Matthias Rath, M.D. have shown through extensive research that a deficiency of vitamin C in the body will speed up the process of arteriosclerosis mainly because it causes defects in the arterial walls due to reduced collagen synthesis. They have shown that vitamin C supplementation in fact can reverse arteriosclerosis.

Vitamin C: A High Powered Antioxidant

Dr. Miller proposes that you take 1,000 to 4,000 milligrams a day to help reduce the oxidation of LDL and prevent heart disease. Usually any form of vitamin C is efficient, but Dr Miller recommends the Ester-C form because it is non-acidic and less irritating to the bowels than the acid form.

The U.S. Recommended Dietary Allowance (RDA) of vitamin C is not nearly enough. In an animal study, it was found that the RDA of vitamin C offered virtually no protection against arterial damage. However when the amount of vitamin C was increased to a dose equivalent to 2,800 mg for a 154 pound (68kg) person, the damage was reversed.

Vitamin C (ascorbic acid) prevents the formation of oxysterols and by combining the amino acid lysine with vitamin C, it may be possible to dissolve clots in the bloodstream. Vitamin C is also required for collagen synthesis and is therefore necessary to maintain the integrity of the walls of arteries.

Dr Cowden says: *"Vitamin C reverses oxidation and prevents free-radical formation. In a diet that involves reducing fats, vitamin C is an integral part of helping the body to repair itself."*

Dr. Cowden recommends that:

- People with existing heart disease take vitamin C and increase the dose up to the level of bowel tolerance in other words keep on increasing the intake to the maximum amount before causing loose stools or diarrhoea.

- Take 3-4 doses daily, increasing the amount until reaching bowel tolerance and to stay on that level (bowel tolerance) until cardiovascular disease is resolved and then go back to a maintenance dose of 3,000 mg daily.

- For prevention of cardiovascular disease take 3,000-10,000 mg daily.

- Higher doses of vitamin C should always be taken with adequate amounts of water, magnesium, and vitamin B6.

Vitamin C: Beneficial for Cholesterol Levels

Many population-based and clinical studies have shown the following:

- There is a direct correlation between the levels of vitamin C levels in a person's body and total cholesterol and HDL cholesterol levels.

- The higher the vitamin C content of the blood,

  - The lower the total cholesterol and triglyceride levels and the higher the HDL cholesterol level.

  - The positive effects on HDL levels were very impressive. For each 0.5 mg/dL raise in vitamin C levels, there is a 14.9 mg/dL in women and 2.1 mg/dL in men, rise in HDL cholesterol. Remember, for every 1% increase in HDL cholesterol the risk of heart disease drops 4%.

  - But the best effect of high-dosage vitamin C is the fact that it reduces the level Lp(a) and its antioxidant activity.

  - The studies also proved that vitamin C supplementation increases HDL levels even if they follow healthy diets.

Note: *According to W. Lee Cowden, M.D., high amounts of the ascorbic acid form of vitamin C taken over a prolonged period of time can leach calcium and other minerals out of the teeth, bones, and other tissues. He recommends that high amounts of ascorbic acid be balanced by mineral ascorbates containing magnesium, potassium, zinc, and manganese.*

Vitamin E: The Inflammation Fighter

Vitamin E is another powerful antioxidant.

The World Health Organization also conducted a study amongst the people of 16 European nations and found that those with low levels of vitamin E were at greater risk for heart disease than those with high blood pressure and high cholesterol levels.

Dr. Miller recommends a dose of 800 IU (international units) per day as the perfect amount to prevent oxidizing of cholesterol. He recommends that we should be using natural, not synthetic vitamin E supplements which contain mixed tocopherols; the label should specify the ingredients alpha-, beta-, and gamma-tocopherol. *"A mix of tocopherols, not just one, is the way vitamin E is found in nature,"* he says.

Vitamin E dissolves in fat and therefore its antioxidant properties get to the places in the body where it can be most effective (the fat) helping to prevent abnormal blood clot formation. Dr. Passwater says that any nutrient that prevents the oxidation of cholesterol such as vitamin E, beta carotene, and coenzyme Q 10 offers a protective factor.

The findings of two studies, both at Harvard Medical School, about the benefits of using Vitamin E published in the New England Journal of Medicine suggest that it:

- Stops platelet aggregation and repairs the lining cells of blood vessels.

- Adds much to the prevention of heart disease in both men and women. The first study involved a group of 87,245 female nurse; The finding was that those who took 100 IU of vitamin E daily for more than two years had a 46% lower risk of heart disease. The second study involved 39,910 male health professionals; The finding was that with daily supplementation of 100 IU of vitamin E heart disease was reduced by 37%

Note: Dr W. Lee Cowden, M.D. Says: *"High dosages of vitamin E are not recommended for people with hypertension, rheumatic heart disease, or ischemic heart disease except under close medical supervision. However, in hypertensive or ischemic heart disease patients, if the dose of vitamin E is raised gradually, the*

blood pressure will usually not rise significantly and there will not
be a greater workload placed on the heart.

Niacin Vitamin B3 – Better than any statin

Dr Mark Stengler, N.D., a naturopathic physician in San Diego
says: "Niacin is a B vitamin that works powerfully to lower LDL
cholesterol."

He goes on to say: *"In my experience, this vitamin is as effective as
any cholesterol-lowering drug on the market."*

Niacin (vitamin B3) lowers cholesterol levels and diminishes the
risk of heart disease and increases the lifespan of people who
suffered a heart attack.

In one study, more than 8,000 middle-aged men who had suffered
heart attacks were given supplements of niacin, estrogen, thyroid
hormone, or a placebo. The results showed that only niacin was
beneficial in lowering the death rate and increasing longevity.

*Dr. Abram Hoffer, M.D., Ph.D., of Victoria, British Columbia,
Canada, saw a patient in 1992 who was a pilot and had not been
able to fly since 1985 because of heart problems. Dr. Hoffer put
him on niacin (3 g daily) and, after 18 months, he was given a
clean bill of health and was able to fly again.*

Another of Dr. Hoffer's patients came to him 20 years ago with angina pectoris. This patient was also treated with niacin and, according to Dr. Hoffer, has had no signs of angina since.

Dr. Stengler recommends taking 1,500 milligrams of niacin a day in the form of inositol hexanicotinate. This form doesn't cause the tingling, itchy, hot rush of blood into the face and upper body. He recommends starting with 500 mg increasing the dose by 500 mg a week until you reach the full amount.

Niacin could have side effects

Conventional physicians are reluctant to prescribe niacin despite the fact that it has proven to be more effective than statins. This is mostly because of the widespread misconception that niacin is a difficult and somewhat dangerous medicine. There is also a lot of confusion about the benefits and the risks for patients who take niacin.

I find it ironic that physicians are "on alert" about the "risks" of niacin but at the same time they are oblivious to the considerable risks and limited benefits of statins as a cholesterol- lowering agent.

One explanation is obviously the fact that niacin is available as a generic supplement which can not be patented by any of the pharmaceutical companies and therefore they can't make money out of it. As a result, niacin is not advertised as widely as the other drugs. Regardless of the advantages of niacin, it accounts for only 7.9% of all cholesterol-lowering prescriptions handed out by conventional practitioners.

The cholesterol-lowering benefits of niacin were first described in the 1950s. It is a well known 'secret' that niacin not only lowers the total cholesterol level but it lowers LDL cholesterol, Lp(a), triglyceride, and fibrinogen (a blood protein that causes clot formation) levels, while at the same time it raises HDL cholesterol levels.

During a study called "The Coronary Drug Project" it was established that niacin was the only cholesterol-lowering agent that actually reduces overall mortality. In a follow up study 15 years later it also showed that the effects are long-term:

- Long-term death rate for patients treated with niacin was actually 11% lower than that of the placebo group,

- Even though the patients were no longer taking the niacin, they still had a lower death rate.

- On the flip side, patients treated with drugs such as clofibrate and/or cholestyramine actually experienced an increased death rate.

- Clofibrate was associated with a 36% higher mortality rate.

- Both clofibrate and cholestyramine lowered cholesterol levels and reduced the mortality rate for coronary artery disease but increased the risk of dying prematurely from cancer, complications of gallbladder surgery (clofibrate causes gallstones), and other conditions.

Clofibrate and cholestyramine have been replaced by new drugs such as lovastatin (Mevacor), pravastatin (Pravochol), simvastatin (Zocor), and gemfibrozil (Lopid) and we already know that the new drugs have not improved much on the side effects that consumers suffer.

Lovastatin vs. Niacin

The Encyclopedia of Natural Medicine Revised 2nd Edition reports as follows:

In 1994, the Annals of Internal Medicine published the first clinical study that directly compared niacin and lovastatin.

The twenty-six-week study was performed at five clinics and involved 136 patients who had coronary heart disease and LDL cholesterol levels greater than 160 mg/dL, and/or more than two coronary heart disease risk factors, or an LDL cholesterol level greater than 190 mg/dL without coronary heart disease or with few coronary heart disease risk factors.

Patients were first placed on a four-week diet, after which eligible patients were randomly assigned to receive treatment with either lovastatin (20 mg/day) or niacin (1.5 g/day).

On the basis of the LDL cholesterol response and patient tolerance, the doses were sequentially increased after ten and eighteen weeks of treatment, to 40 and 80 mg/day of lovastatin or 3 and 4.5 g/day of niacin, respectively.

In the two patient groups, sixty-six percent of patients treated with lovastatin, and fifty-four percent of patients treated with niacin.

The results indicated that, while lovastatin produced a greater reduction in LDL cholesterol levels, niacin provided better overall results despite the fact that fewer patients were able to tolerate a full dosage of niacin because of skin flushing.

The percentage increase in HDL cholesterol, a more significant indicator for coronary heart disease, was dramatically in favor of niacin (thirty three percent versus seven percent).

Equally as impressive was the percentage decrease in Lp(a) level with niacin treatment.

While niacin produced a thirty-five-percent reduction in Lp(a) levels, lovastatin did not produce any effect. Niacin's effect on Lp(a) in this study confirmed a previous study that showed that niacin (4 grams/day) reduced Lp(a) levels by thirty-eight percent.

In another study it was shown that niacin raised the level of HDL cholesterol by 30% while gemfibrozil raised it by 10% and lovastatin by 6%.

Dealing with the Side Effects of Niacin

The most common and bothersome side effect of niacin is the skin flushing that typically occurs 20-30 minutes after consumption. Other occasional and rare side effects of niacin include gastric irritation, nausea, and liver damage.

Niacin can also harm blood sugar control and should therefore always be used with close observation in patients with diabetes. Niacin should not be used by patients with pre-existing liver disease or elevated levels of liver enzymes. For these patient groups, gugulipid (an extract of Commiphora mukul), garlic, or pantethine is recommended. See the herbs section for more details about gugulipid and garlic.

The safest form of niacin is known as inositol hexaniacinate. This form of niacin has been used in Europe for a long time to lower cholesterol levels and improve blood flow. It provides slightly better results than standard niacin and is much better tolerated, in other words less flushing.

How to take Niacin - Some Practical Recommendations

- Tell your physician that you are taking niacin and that you wish to be monitored.

- Once on niacin (any form) get your liver functions and cholesterol levels checked every 3 months.

- Always take niacin with meals.

- Niacin should be considered the first cholesterol-lowering agent to try.

- Most side effects like skin flushing and other can be avoided by using inositol hexaniacinate.

- Do not use sustained-release niacin at all.

- If pure crystalline niacin is used, start with a dose of 100 mg three times per day, and carefully increase the dosage over a period of four to six weeks to the full therapeutic dose of 1.5 g to 3 g daily in divided doses.

- If inositol hexaniacinate is being used, begin with 500 mg three times per day for two weeks, then increase to 1,000 mg for 2 weeks and then increase to 1,500 mg.

Pantethine aka as Vitamin B5 or Coenzyme A

Pantethine is the best and most effective compound to lower blood triglyceride levels.

Pantethine is the stable form of pantetheine or the active form of vitamin B5, or pantothenic acid also the most important component of coenzyme A (CoA).

CoA is engaged in conveying of fats to and from the body cells, without CoA the cells of our body would not be able to utilize fats as energy.

It has been shown that pantethine can significantly lower cholesterol but on the other hand pantothenic acid has very little (if any) effect in lowering cholesterol and triglyceride levels.

Pantethine at the standard dose of 900 mg (300 mg 3 times) per day can:

- Reduce triglyceride levels up to 32%.

- Reduce total cholesterol levels up to 19%.

- Reduce LDL cholesterol levels up to 21%.

- Increase HDL cholesterol levels up to 23%

To date no toxicity or side effects from taking pantethine has been reported.

Vitamin B6 – Prevents Heart Attacks and Stroke

There is a large body of scientific research and evidence to prove the efficiencies of vitamin B6 (pyridoxine). It is also safe and inexpensive.

B6 helps the body to resist the arterial damage and platelet aggregation that speeds up the onset of heart disease. It also converts homocysteine to the harmless chemical cystathionine, and therefore helps to prevent the oxidation of cholesterol.

Interest in the connection between vitamin B6 and heart disease began when a heart researcher, Dr Kilmer S. McCully, M.D., discovered that people with heart disease had almost 80% less B6 levels than healthy individuals. He also discovered that people who suffered from a heart attack or angina recovered very quickly when given 200 mg of B6 daily combined with a low-fat, mostly vegetarian diet.

In 1949, Dr Moses M. Suzman, M.D., a South African neurologist and internist, conducted extensive research on a large group of people who showed signs of arterial damage. He placed them on 100 mg of vitamin B6 per day, while patients who had already had heart attacks or angina were given 200 mg per day. In addition, the patients with the most serious conditions were given folic acid (5 mg), vitamin E (100- 600 IU), magnesium, and zinc.

The results were astonishing. The patients recovered quickly with their angina and other heart related problems diminishing dramatically or disappeared. However, those who dropped out of his treatment program soon found their cardiac problems returning.

Coenzyme Q10

More than 50 years ago, Karl Folkers, Ph.D., a biomedical scientist at the University of Texas, in Austin, discovered that coenzyme Q10 helps to strengthen the heart muscles.

Since then studies have revealed that CoQ10 protect against atherosclerosis and have antioxidant properties that may protect against the formation of oxysterols.

Dr. Gordon reports that he had outstanding success using supplements of CoQ10, amino acids, and herbs to help infants avoid risky surgery. He says: *"In one case I went to see a newborn diagnosed with myocardiopathy, a disease of the heart muscle. With the family's permission, I treated the baby with coenzyme Q10, carnitine [an amino acid], magnesium, vitamin C, a multivitamin/mineral formula, liquid garlic, and hawthorn berry extract. The baby recovered without the heart transplant surgery that was being recommended by the university medical center."*

Coenzyme Q10 (CoQ10) is produced in the body and is vital for the basic functioning of cells. Research has shown that CoQ10 levels are low in people with chronic diseases such as heart conditions, muscular dystrophies, Parkinson's disease, cancer, diabetes, and HIV/AIDS. Levels of CoQ10 in the body can be increased by taking CoQ10 supplements.

On his website at www.thenutritionreporter.com/coenzymeq10.html Jack Challem discusses the importance of CoQ10 and heart disease as follows:

Heart disease. Cancer. AIDS. As unbelievable as it might sound, each of these deadly diseases often responds to a coenzyme Q10, a little known nutrient that can make a big difference in your health.

Granted, such "cure all" statements leave people wondering whether CoQ10 is just the latest panacea of the month. Rest assured: the benefits of this nutrient are well documented in the medical journals. It's one of the most frequently prescribed heart "drugs" in Japan and widely used in Europe-and one company even owns the patent for the CoQ10 treatment of AIDS.

Ask your doctor about CoQ10, though, and he'll probably say he's never heard of it. Part of the problem is CoQ10's name. "Most doctors don't know what a coenzyme is," said Karl Folkers, Ph.D., one of the researchers who pioneered CoQ10. Most biochemists know it as ubiquinone, an equally arcane name.

CoQ10 is a little easier to appreciate when you remember that vitamins function as co-enzymes in the body, furthering thousands of essential biochemical reactions. CoQ10's key role is in producing adenosine triphosphate (ATP), needed for energy production in every cell of the body. Secondary to that, CoQ10 functions as a powerful antioxidant.

This vitamin-like nutrient occurs widely in the food supply, though not always in significant amounts. In addition, each cell in the body manufactures CoQ10, though not always very efficiently. That means you may not be getting enough for optimal health.

"Like the vitamins discovered in the early part of this century, CoQ10 is an essential element of food that can now be used medicinally," explained Peter Langsjoen, M.D., a cardiologist in Tyler, Texas.

CoQ10 and the Heart

CoQ10 was discovered in 1957-relatively late as vitamins discoveries occur, by Frederick Crane, Ph.D., now at Purdue University in Indiana. Four years later, Peter D. Mitchell, Ph.D., of the University of Edinburgh, figured out how CoQ10 produces energy at the cellular level and, in 1978, won the Nobel Prize for chemistry for this discovery.

By the mid-1960s, Japanese researchers recognized that CoQ10 concentrated in the myocardium, or heart muscle. Its role in the heart makes sense: the heart, one of the body's most energetic organs, beats approximately 100,000 times a day and 36 million times a year, and depends on CoQ10 for "bioenergetics." In the early 1980s, Folkers, director of the Institute for Biochemical

Research at the University of Texas, and the late Per H. Langsjoen, M.D. (Peter's father), conducted the first study of CoQ10 in the treatment of cardiomyopathy, a form of progressive heart failure.

The findings were astounding. In a well-controlled study, 19 patients who were expected to die from heart failure rebounded with an "extraordinary clinical improvement," according to Folkers and Langsjoen's report in the Proceedings of the National Academy of Sciences of the USA (June 1985;82: 4240-4).

Case studies demonstrate the dramatic effect of CoQ10. In Biochemical and Biophysical Research Communications (Jan 15, 1993;182:247-53), Folkers described a 43-year-old man suffering from cardiomyopathy. After being given CoQ10, his enlarged heart became smaller (indicating it was working more efficiently), and he was able to resume an "extremely active athletic lifestyle." The heart function of another patient, a 50-year-old man with very severe cardiomyopathy, returned after he took CoQ10, and he has since had "no limitations of activity."

Numerous other studies have confirmed the role of CoQ10 in treating heart failure, which is otherwise treated with drugs (such as beta blockers and ACE inhibitors)-or with a heart transplant. A sampling:

- *Sixty-five cardiologists treating 806 patients for heart failure or ischemic heart disease indicated "significant" benefits from CoQ10. (Langsjoen, PH, Klinische Wochenschrift, 1988;66:583-90.)*

- *Twenty-five hundred heart failure patients at 173 Italian medical centers were given 50 to 150 mg CoQ10 daily for three months. Eighty percent of the patients had some type of improvement. (Clinical Investigator, Aug. 1993;71S:145-9)*

- *A 12-month double-blind study compared 319 patients taking CoQ10 with 322 taking a placebo. CoQ10 reduced complications of heart failure as well as the need for hospitalization. (Clinical Investigator, Aug. 1993;71S:134-6).*

Therapeutic dosages of CoQ10 for serious diseases range from 200-400 mg. daily, ideally under a physician's supervision. It works in diverse conditions because the basic underlying mechanisms are the same-energy production at the cellular level and antioxidant protection against free radicals. In an interview, Folkers said that CoQ10 is safe and has no negative side effects, though it may decrease the need for other heart medicines. A common preventive dose ranges from 10-30 mg daily.

Vitamin B12, Folic Acid, Selenium & Beta Carotene

Vitamin B12

It has been proven that low levels of vitamin B12 go hand in hand with high levels of homocysteine levels and as soon as B12 levels rise, homocysteine levels decrease. It is recommended that you get a blood test to determine your B12 levels.

Folic Acid

By now I am sure that we are all well aware of the need to get the levels of homocysteine down as low as possible. Recent studies proved that the intake of vitamins B6, B12, and folic acid dramatically lowers the levels of homocysteine in the body.

A Three Pronged Attack with Selenium

Selenium is a trace mineral which has been shown to be very beneficial in the fight against cholesterol:

- It increases the levels of glutathione.

- It lowers LDL.

- It increases HDL

Dr. Miller says: *"Selenium is absolutely critical to any cholesterol-lowering program."* He recommends a daily multivitamin that contains at least 200 micrograms of selenium. Furthermore is an antioxidant which also reduces platelet aggregation.

Beta Carotene

Researchers at Johns Hopkins University; in Baltimore, Maryland, found that people who have the highest levels of beta carotene were 50% less likely to attract heart disease than those with the lower levels.

Dr. Cowden recommends that you take mixed carotenoids rather than beta carotene alone. Beta carotene is also found in abundance in yellow vegetables like carrots and pumpkin.

Magnesium, Zinc, Copper, Calcium, Chromium & Potassium

Magnesium

It has been found that people who die of sudden heart attacks have very low levels of magnesium and potassium compared to those who don't.

It has been found that magnesium plays an extremely important role in maintaining a healthy heart:

- It helps to widen arteries and ease the heart's pumping of blood, thus preventing arrhythmias (irregular heartbeats).

- It prevents calcification of the blood vessels.

- It also lowers total cholesterol, raise HDL cholesterol, and inhibit platelet aggregation.

Dr. Cowden says it is not a matter of just taking magnesium supplements *"Most doctors don't use the best form for optimum absorption. It's more effective to use magnesium malate, glycinate, taurate, or aspartate, or even herbal magnesium such as red raspberry, but some patients need intravenous or intramuscular magnesium to quickly raise their magnesium to ideal levels."* Magnesium oxide should not be used.

Dr. Alan R. Gaby, M.D., former President of the American Holistic Medical Association, discovered that cases of congestive heart failure respond well to an intravenous injection of a "cocktail" composed of magnesium chloride hexahydrate, hydroxocobalamin, pyridoxine hydrochloride, dexpanthenol, B-complex vitamins, and vitamin C.

Zinc and Copper

Dr Amy Rothenberg, N.D., a naturopathic physician in Enfield, Connecticut says: "Zinc and copper increase HDL and reduce LDL." He recommends 30 milligrams of zinc and 1 to 2 milligrams of copper daily, as part of a multivitamin/mineral supplement.

Calcium

Calcium has been shown to decrease total cholesterol and inhibit platelet aggregation. Dr. Cowden recommends that herbal forms of calcium are more effective for heart disease patients.

Chromium

Low levels of chromium have been linked to heart disease by several studies. It has been shown to also lower total cholesterol and triglycerides and raise HDL cholesterol and is even more effective in lowering cholesterol when combined with niacin (vitamin B3).

Potassium

Hypertension (high blood pressure) is often present in people with heart disease. Potassium can help decrease a patient's dependence on blood pressure medication or diuretic drugs which all have nasty side effects.

Amino Acids

The amino acid L-arginine, has been shown to lower blood pressure and supplementation with L-arginine immediately after a heart attack can help damaged heart muscle expand again. In one study, L-carnitine, given orally (2,000 mg daily for 28 days), improved the condition of 51 patients who had undergone heart attacks showing that the amount of damaged heart muscle after 28 days was significantly less, the incidence of angina and arrhythmia was reduced by 50%.

Proanthocyanidin (PCA)

Dr. Passwater, says *"Pycnogenol, an antioxidant derived from maritime pine bark or a comparable PCA extract from grape seeds, enhances heart health by protecting LDL cholesterol from oxidation and by protecting the integrity of the artery lining. In addition PCA helps keep the blood platelets from becoming stickier and developing a tendency to unnecessarily clump together"*

Vitamins and Minerals Treatment Summary

Below are some guidelines of dosage and frequency, but please note that the consumption of Vitamins and Minerals should be discussed with your health professional to determine the right quantities, timings and other factors suiting your personal circumstances.

Where applicable I have divided the treatment recommendations into 2 sections: Therapeutic (to be taken when you have heart disease or high cholesterol) and Preventive (to be taken when you try to prevent heart disease or high cholesterol).

Vitamin C is the first line of defense and attack

<u>Therapeutic</u>

Take vitamin C and increase the dose up to the level of bowel tolerance. In other words keep on increasing the intake to the maximum amount before causing loose stools or diarrhoea. This could be as high as 10,000 mg per day. Take 3-4 doses daily.

<u>Prevention</u>

Take 3,000- 5,000 mg daily. Remember higher doses of vitamin C should always be taken with adequate amounts of water, magnesium, and vitamin B6.

Vitamin E is the inflammation fighter

The name Vitamin E refers to two different chemical substances tocopherol and tocotrienol. The most common form in use today is the form of Vitamin E that contains tocopherol and has always been regarded as the best (most powerful) form to use.

However, lately, scientists found that Vitamin E containing tocotrienol is in fact 30 to 60 times more powerful than the one containing tocopherol.

- Dr. Miller recommends a dose of 800 IU (international units) per day of vitamin E supplements which contain mixed tocopherols; the label should specify the ingredients alpha-, beta-, and gamma-tocopherol.

- Dr Donald Carrow M. D., founder and director of the Florida Institute of Health in Tampa, recommends that if you take Vitamin E containing tocotrienol you should look for one that includes a mix of tocotrienols called alpha, beta, and gamma. You should take 50mg 3 times per day.

Niacin Vitamin B3 – Better than any statin

Please make sure that you read and understand all the information about Niacin I have given you before. Do not take Niacin without supervision of a health professional and make sure you go for regular tests as recommended before.

Only use the form of Niacin called inositol hexaniacinate. Do not use sustained-release niacin at all.

With inositol hexaniacinate, begin with 500 mg three times per day for two weeks, then increase to 1,000 mg for 2 weeks and then increase to 1,500 mg.

Pantethine

300 mg 3 times per day.

Vitamin B6

Therapeutic

200 mg per day

Prevention

100 mg per day

Coenzyme Q10

Therapeutic

200-400 mg. daily, ideally under a physician's supervision

Prevention

Common preventive dose ranges from 10-30 mg daily.

Vitamin B12, Folic Acid, Selenium & Beta Carotene As directed on the labels except for selenium you should take 200 mcg (micro grams) per day.

Magnesium, Zinc, Copper, Calcium, Chromium & Potassium
Take 1,000 mg of magnesium (500 mg twice a day) and take a multivitamin containing Zinc, Copper, Calcium, Chromium and Potassium.

Proanthocyanidin (PCA)

As directed on the label.

Alternative Treatment - Herbal Remedies

It is always best to consult a skilled herbalist before taking herbs.

David L. Hoffman, B.Sc., M.N.I.M.H., of Sebastopol, California, past President of the American Herbalists Guild says: *"Some herbs have a potent and direct impact on the heart itself, such as Digitalis purpurea (foxglove), and form the basis of drug therapy for heart failure."*

Hoffman recommends a "heart tonic" consisting of an equal amount of:

- Tinctures of hawthorn berries, Ginkgo biloba, and linden flowers (1/2 teaspoon three times a day).

- He also suggests the addition of tincture of motherwort to prevent palpitations and garlic to help manage cholesterol.

Hawthorn Berry

The extract from hawthorn berry has been described as one of the most promising herbal remedies for the treatment of heart disease. It has been found to improve the circulation of blood to the heart by dilating (widening) the blood vessels and relieving spasms of the arterial walls.

Dr. Gordon says: *"Hawthorn berry may render unnecessary medications that decrease the rate and force of heart contraction in the treatment of heart disease, as it performs a similar function to these drugs."*

Ginger and Olive Leafs

Ginger has been shown to have many healing benefits. Ginger lowers cholesterol levels and makes the blood platelets less sticky.

Extracts from olive leaves lower blood pressure and working against free-radical activity the leaf also contains natural vitamin C and biofiavonoids, such as rutin, luteolin, and hesperidin, which are needed for maintenance of the capillary walls.

Garlic

The sulfur in garlic is an antioxidant and also helps to dissolve clots. Garlic lowers blood pressure and cholesterol levels.

Garlic has proven to be one of the most beneficial herbs available to mankind for many health conditions. Here I will focus on the benefits it has for heart disease.

Fresh garlic contains 0.1% to 0.36% of a volatile oil (also called essential oil) composed of sulfur-containing compounds, one of the compounds, allicin, is the one which is responsible for the smell. Unfortunately, allicin is also the component with the strong medicinal properties.

The garlic essential oil consists of about 60% allicin when it is fresh. However, once garlic has been cooked it looses much of the allicin in the essential oil.

Therefore the real benefit of garlic is obtained when eating fresh garlic. However, there are commercial preparations which we can use that will bring the same benefits as fresh garlic.

Commercial Garlic Preparations

In order to realize the positive effect of garlic from commercial preparations you should make sure it contains a sufficient dosage of allicin.

Many of the commercial preparations provide odorless garlic which is obviously more "socially acceptable." Based on a great deal of clinical research, the recommendation is that a commercial garlic product should provide a daily dose of at least 4,000 mcg of allicin which is the equivalent of eating 4,000 mg or 4 cloves of garlic per day.

Manufacturers of garlic products promote their product as the best, but how do we know who to believe? The best product is the one that is rich in all garlic compounds and most resembles fresh garlic.

What about aged garlic? Research has shown that aged garlic does not provide the required allicin levels that compares with the equivalent of 4,000 mg of fresh garlic.

The Encyclopedia of Natural Medicine Revised 2nd Edition reports that significantly better results are achieved in a shorter amount of time with the fresh garlic preparations compared to aged garlic.

Similarly, blood pressure reductions have also been greater when using fresh garlic instead of aged garlic. With fresh garlic preparations, typical reductions of 11 mm Hg for the systolic and 5.0 in the diastolic are usually achieved within a one- to three month period.

Garlic and Heart Disease

It has been proven that it may not be necessary to take garlic supplements if the dietary intake of garlic and onion can be increased.

Guggul: Another Excellent Cholesterol-Lowering Herb

Dr Virender Sodhi, M.D. (Ayurved), N.D., an Ayurvedic and naturopathic physician and director of the American School of Ayurvedic Sciences in Bellevue, Washington says: *"I have dramatically reduced LDL cholesterol and increased HDL cholesterol with just this one herb,"*

Gugulipid is an extract of the mukul myrrh tree (Commiphora mukul), native to India. The active components of gugulipid are guggulsterone and E-guggulsterone.

Several studies have shown that gugulipid has an ability to lower both cholesterol and triglyceride levels quite significantly.

- Total cholesterol levels dropped between 14% and 27% in 4-12 weeks.

- LDL dropped between 25% and 35% and triglyceride dropped between 22% and 30%

- HDL cholesterol levels increased between 16% and 20%.

Gugulipid is without side effects and has been shown to be safe to use during pregnancy.

Gugulipid lowers cholesterol by increasing the liver's metabolism of LDL cholesterol. It has been shown to prevent atherosclerosis and aid in the regression of preexisting atherosclerotic plaques as well as a mild effect in inhibiting platelet aggregation. The dosage of gugulipid is based on its guggulsterone content. Clinical studies have demonstrated that gugulipid extract, standardized to contain 25mg of guggulsterone per 500 mg tablet, given three times per day, is an effective treatment for elevated cholesterol levels, elevated triglyceride levels, or both.

Once your cholesterol levels are back to normal, Dr. Sodhi recommends reducing the dosage to 300 milligrams a day.

Herbal Treatment Summary

It is highly recommended that you do not embark on herbal treatments without the help of a qualified herbalist. Furthermore, you should inform your physician of the herbs that you take.

- **Flaxseed oil:** 1 tablespoon daily

- **Niacin** (as inositol hexaniacinate): 500 mg three times per day with meals for two weeks, then increase dosage to 1,000 mg three times per day with meals and increase to 1,500 mg three times per day after 2 months.

- **Garlic:** minimum of 4,000 mcg of allicin per day

- **Gugulipid** extract, standardized to contain 25 mg of guggulsterone per 500 mg tablet, 3 times per day. Once your cholesterol levels are back to normal reduce the dosage to 300 mg per day.

If you follow the recommendations above you could expect to see the following results within the first two months:

- Reduction in total cholesterol level of 50 to 75 mg/dL where initial total cholesterol levels were above 250 mg/dl.

- In cases where the initial cholesterol level is above 300 mg/dL, it may take 4-6 months before cholesterol levels begin to reach recommended levels.

Once the cholesterol is below 200 mg/dl, reduce the dosage of niacin to 500 mg three times per day for two months. If the cholesterol levels creep up above 200 mg/dL, then raise the dosage of niacin back to 1,000 mg three times per day. If the cholesterol level remains below 200 mg/dL, then withdraw the niacin completely and check the cholesterol levels in two months. Reinstitute niacin therapy if levels creep up over 200 mg/dL.

Garlic and flaxseed oil supplementation can be continued indefinitely, if desired. Gugulipid can be added to the above protocol if, after four months, the total cholesterol level remains above 2 mg/dL. Gugulipid is also suitable for the rare patient who cannot tolerate inositol hexaniacinate.

Alternative Treatments for Angina

It is worth repeating what I said before: Angina is a sign of heart disease! It has been described as the edge of a cliff and you need guidance (medical treatment) away from it. Those angina pains are the messengers from the future!

If you have been suffering from angina attacks, chances are that you are already taking a prescription drug such as nitroglycerin (Nitrolingual) to keep your angina attacks under control. Usually it is recommended that you place 1 tablet of nitroglycerin under the tongue every 5 minutes until the pain is gone and not taking more than 3 tablets. If the pain does not subside after 3 tablets or 15 minutes you should get someone to take you to the nearest hospital as a matter of extreme urgency. The nitroglycerine is very effective at opening up the arteries allowing more oxygen to come through to the heart muscle. However, as with all conventional drugs and treatments it only treats the symptoms and does not address the problem of why the angina attack happened in the first place.

Alternative practitioners therefore recommend that you combine the intake of nutritional supplements with prescription drugs to help reduce and liberate you of angina attacks. A regimen of natural supplements will improve blood flow to the heart muscle, says Dr. Julian Whitaker M.D. founder and director of the Whitaker Wellness Institute in Newport Beach California.

Coenzyme Q10: Will Revitalize the Heart

Ask any alternative practitioner what is the best remedy for treating angina and they will tell you that nothing beats coenzyme Q10 (Co Q10). It is a natural substance found in every cell of the body as vital for our existence as oxygen. We cannot live without Co Q10 as it is essential for the manufacturing of the energy that powers the cells of the body and the heart muscle.

Dr Stephen T. Sinatra, M.D., is a cardiologist and director of the New England Heart Center in Manchester, Connecticut and he highly recommends CO Q10 and says that a study showed that people with angina who were taking CoQ10 could decrease their nitroglycerin intake.

He treats his angina patients with a daily dose of 90 to 180 mg of CO Q10 taken with or after meals. He also says that there are no significant adverse effects from CO Q10 and people can take it for the rest of their lives.

See the previous sections for more information about Co Q10.

Carnitine: Enhances the Effect of Co Q10

Dr Michael Janson, M.D., consultant physician at Path to Health in Burlington, Massachusetts suggests it has been shown that the intake of carnitine (a vitamin-like amino acid) in combination with Co Q10, are more likely to reduce angina pain and the frequency as opposed to only taking Co Q10.

Dr. Janson advises his angina patients to take Co Q10 and 500 to 1,000 milligrams of carnitine 2 or 3 or even 4 times a day, depending on the severity and frequency of their angina.

Pantethine: Lowers Cholesterol as well

Pantethine, also known as coenzyme A, inhibits cholesterol synthesis and has been shown in clinical trials to dramatically reduce cholesterol and has been proven very effective against angina. See the previous sections for more information about pantethine.

Vitamin E (Tocotrienol): Potent Heart Attack Protection

Dr Donald Carrow, M.D., founder and director of the Florida Institute of Health in Tampa says there can be no doubt that Vitamin E can help prevent or reverse heart disease this has been proven over and over again in many studies

Tocotrienol is a super powerful form of vitamin E says Dr Carrow. He believes that it is 30 to 60 times more powerful than vitamin E containing tocopherol-which obviously makes it one of the best ways to treat and reverse angina.

It is believed that tocotrienols act like a blood-thinning drug helping to stop the formation of blood clots where arteries are clogged.

Dr. Carrow prescribes for his angina patients 50 mg of mixed tocotrienols (a product that includes forms of tocotrienols called alpha, beta, delta, and gamma) three times a day.

Magnesium Citrate: Improves Blood Flow Immediately

It has been proven that magnesium citrate opens the arteries of the heart and strengthens the heart muscle. Always remember that magnesium deficiency plays a significant role in angina.

However, it must be remembered that magnesium citrate is a laxative and taking too much will upset the stomach. Dr Carrow recommends that people with angina take 1 ounce (28 grams) of magnesium citrate which is a non-laxative dose once a day on an empty stomach.

Dr. Carrow says it has been found that taking an extra 1 ounce (28 grams) dose of magnesium citrate during a minor angina attack stop the attack.

It is important to talk to your doctor before using magnesium citrate for angina and it is also very important to never use it as a substitute for any drug treatment.

Homeopathy: Cactus can Stop the Pain Fast

Mark Stengler, N.D. a naturopathic physician in San Diego says this is a remedy used by homeopaths that has proven to work well to stop the pain of an angina attack. He prescribes 30C strength of the medicine, dissolving two pellets in the mouth every 5 minutes until the pain is gone.

Again it is very important to note that homeopathic Cactus must not be taken instead of any drugs prescribed by a physician but should be taken with it.

Prinzmetal's Variant Angina

This type of angina is not related to narrowed arteries caused by buildup of plaque (atherosclerosis) but is rather caused by a spasm of one of the coronary arteries. This spasm usually happens while a person is in a resting position e.g. lying down, sitting or at odd times during the day.

This type of angina responds very well to magnesium supplementation.

Angina Prevention Supplement Treatment Summary

- Coenzyme Q10 – 150 -300 mg per day

- L-carnitine 500 mg 3 times per day

- Pantethine – 300 mg 3 times per day

- Magnesium bound to citrate or aspartate – 200-400 mg per day

- Vitamin E - 50 mg of mixed tocotrienols 3 times per day

- Carnitine 500 to 1,000 milligrams of 2,or 3 or even 4 times a day, depending on the severity and frequency of their angina.

A Warm Shower Might Ease the Pain

Dr Donald Carrow says; *"Taking a very warm shower or bath dilates blood vessels throughout your body, including the arteries leading to the heart. This can help stop the pain of repeated episodes of minor angina.*

I tell all of my patients with angina to take very warm showers or baths when they're having minor attacks, and many of them get instant relief.

One caution, however: Be sure that the bathroom has a good exhaust fan, and turn it on before you get in the shower or tub. Steam can reduce the amount of oxygen in a room, making angina worse".

If the angina pain does not go away after 5 to 10 minutes you must go to the nearest hospital urgently.

Again it is important to note that this treatment brings only temporarily relieve and should never take the place of prescribed medications.

Alternative Treatments for Stroke

Strokes are the third largest cause of death in the USA.

Stroke happens when the arteries supplying the brain become blocked, leading to a blocking of the oxygen supply to a portion of the brain. Damage is usually loss of speech, movement, or eyesight.

The standard treatment for victims of stroke is months of physiotherapy sometimes recovering only minimal function.

However German researchers recognized that the loss of functioning of an arm or leg after a stroke was similar to symptoms of the bends," a sometimes fatal affliction deep-sea divers can get from ascending too quickly.

They found that restoring the balance of nitrogen and oxygen in the blood cured divers of the bends, and physicians suspected that victims of stroke might be helped in a similar manner.

Hyperbaric Oxygen Therapy

Scientists have built a hyperbaric oxygen chamber in which they place a patient who had suffered a stroke. Inside the chamber the atmospheric pressure is altered which forces oxygen into the tissues so that it reaches the cells in its most easily utilized state.

Below is an extract from **Alternative Medicine: The Definitive Guide; Second Edition** discussing this therapy in more detail.

According to David Hughes, Ph.D., of the Hyperbaric Oxygen institute, in San Bernardino, California, the treatment has been used quite successfully in Germany. Hyperbaric oxygen therapy increases oxygen to the brain and the increased atmospheric pressure may have therapeutic benefits for swollen tissues.

An infusion of highly diluted hydrogen peroxide into the bloodstream may have the same effect, and hydrogen peroxide has been shown to dissolve lipids from the arterial walls.

Antioxidants

W. Lee Cowden, M.D., found that if patients who suffered a stroke are treated within the first hours after the incident with:

... a combination of high antioxidant intake, essential fatty acids, and either hyperbaric oxygen therapy or body-bag" ozone therapy, then a dramatic regression of stroke symptoms can occur.

Patients regain sensation, strength, and mental clarity, as well as motor and sensory skills and orientation. In his treatment, Dr. Cowden uses the antioxidarns vitamin E, beta carotene, ascorbyl palmitate (a form of vitamin C), and proanthocyanidins (an antioxidant found in maritime pine bark or grape seeds) as well as the essential fatty acids eicosapentaenoic acid (EPA) and docosahexaenoic acid (DHA) to help prevent damage to brain cells.

Biological Therapies

Harvey Bigelsen, M.D., Medical Director of the Center for Progressive Medicine, in Scottsdale, Arizona, uses biological therapies developed by the late German bacteriologist Gunther Enderlein, M.D., Ph.D., to help alleviate the symptoms of stroke.

According to Dr. Bigelsen, Dr. Enderlein theorized that disease must be treated at the cellular level and formulated his remedies accordingly. The remedies are extracts of plants and fungi that, once injected into the patient, work according to the principles of homeopathy.

Dr. Enderlein maintained that bacteria can take on both harmless and harmful forms; by injecting harmless forms of bacteria, those harmful entities in the body will revert to their harmless state.

Dr. Bigelsen uses these remedies intravenously to bring strokes-in-progress to a halt.

One such patient was treated intravenously and within five minutes the crisis of the stroke was broken and the symptoms alleviated. The patient was then treated with cell therapy to stimulate the brain tissue and chelation therapy to help clear out the arteries. He was able to walk out of the hospital with no residual disability and resumed work a few days later.

Low Energy Lasers

Margaret A. Naeser, PhD., Associate Research Professor of Neurology at Boston University School of Medicine, has conducted research on the use of low-energy lasers (20 milliwatt red to infrared laser light) in the treatment of paralysis in stroke.

Five of her six subjects showed improvement and patients with mild-to-moderate paralysis responded better than those with severe paralysis, according to Dr. Naeser. The improvements were observed even when treatments were begun three or four years after the stroke.

David A. Steenblock, M.S., D.O., of Mission Viejo, California, a specialist in alternative treatments (especially hyperbaric oxygen) for stroke, offers the following recommendations for stroke prevention:

- Avoid tobacco smoke and alcohol.

188

- Don't use amphetamines, cocaine, or other illicit drugs as these can be harmful to the heart.

- After age 50, have your carotid arteries checked every five years for atherosclerosis.

- Monitor your blood pressure.

- Exercise daily.

- Eat fresh, non-processed vegetables.

- Eat a high-fiber diet.

- Avoid fats, cholesterol, and sugar and keep your weight down to help prevent diabetes, which affects the heart.

- Take magnesium, calcium, vitamins E and C, and bioflavonoids.

- If you are a woman over 35, avoid birth control pills.

- Quickly correct any medical problems that develop.

Administered according to established protocol, not one serious side effect has ever been reported.

Alternative Treatment - Other Therapies

Don't believe it when you are told that there is only conventional treatment available for heart disease. You have other options which has proved to be more effective than the current conventional methods with all its dangerous side effects.

Below is an extract from Alternative Medicine: The Definitive Guide; Second Edition: Larry Trivieri, JR Editor, Introduced by Burton Goldberg about the various alternatives and their benefits.

Chelation Therapy

There is mounting evidence that chelation therapy offers an alternative to the hundreds of thousands of bypass surgeries and angioplasties performed each year. Chelation therapy is traditionally used to treat poisoning from toxic metals by removing them from the body with a chemical agent. Norman Clarke, Sr., M.D., Director of Research at Providence Hospital, in Detroit, Michigan, hypothesized that since chelation with EDTA (ethylenediaminetetraacetic acid) removed calcium from pipes and boilers, it may be useful to remove calcium plaque in patients with arteriosclerosis. His experiments confirmed his theory, and angina patients treated by Dr. Clarke reported dramatic relief from chest pain.

EDTA chelation therapy has since proven to be safe and effective in the treatment and prevention of ailments linked to atherosclerosis, such as heart attacks, stroke, peripheral vascular disease (leading to pain in the legs and ultimately gangrene), as well as arterial blockages. According to current drug safety standards, aspirin is nearly 31/2 times more toxic than EDTA.

During a chelation therapy session, EDTA is given intravenously to remove plaque and calcium deposits from the arterial walls and then the unwanted material is excreted through the urine. The treatment is usually administered several times per week over a course of two or three months in order to restore complete circulation.

In a 1988 study of 2,870 cases, Efrain Olszewer, M.D., and James Carter, M.D., head of nutrition at the Department of Applied Health Science, School of Public Health and Tropical Medicine, at Tulane University; documented that EDTA chelation therapy brought about significant improvement in 93.9% of patients suffering from coronary artery blockage. Elmer Cranton, M.D., of Troutdale, Virginia, estimates chelation therapy can help avoid bypass surgery in 85% of cases. He points out that during the time that chelation therapy has been administered according to established protocol not one serious side effect has been reported.

Dr. Gordon points out that EDTA chelation can be beneficial for bypass candidates even when the therapy appears unsuccessful in reducing the amount of calcification in coronary arteries. The reason for this, according to Dr. Gordon, has to do with the fact that 85% of heart attacks, strokes, and other types of cardiovascular disease are caused by the rupture of vulnerable, non-calcified arterial plaque and subsequent clot formation.

"It is now widely accepted that the underlying cause of death in heart attacks and strokes is from a blood clot related to this vulnerable, soft or non-calcified, plaque due to an active infection in the arterial wall," Dr. Gordon explains.

"Unfortunately, most patients are unaware of this information about vulnerable plaque or that it is readily detected by currently available vascular tests. As a result, patients who choose chelation therapy instead of bypass are usually disappointed should they learn they still have calcified coronary vessels and may then mistakenly opt for surgery despite the fact that their so—called 'unsuccessful' chelation treatments have enabled them to sustain

a far higher level of physical activity than before treatment." Dr. Gordon adds that improved oxygenation of heart tissues usually results from intravenous chelation. "This, in and of itself is a reasonable goal for patients with cardiovascular conditions," he says.

Because new evidence suggests that most heart attacks and strokes are due to blood clots caused by vulnerable plaque, Dr. Gordon believes that a "carefully and rationally developed" oral chelation formula can be as beneficial as intravenous chelation in helping to prevent such conditions, but in a different manner and without producing the longevity benefits routinely observed with I.V. EDTA. "There appears to be benefits from both therapies," Dr. Gordon says, "but intravenous administration of EDTA cannot permanently reduce inflammation or excessive clotting tendencies. For this reason, most patients believe their I.V. chelation treatments are reversing their arteriosclerosis, yet all too often we are learning that is not the case."

To ensure that his heart patients receive the most comprehensive care, Dr. Gordon developed and employs his own oral chelation protocol. "I have been able to document significant improvements of blood flow to the legs, head, and heart of patients experiencing problems of clot, heart spasm, and arrhythmia with the use of oral chelation, so that fewer than 5% have had to have heart surgery," Dr. Gordon reports. One example of such a patient was a man in his mid-fifties, who came to Dr. Gordon after a series of monthly small, recurring strokes. "An arteriogram revealed that he had bilateral, high- grade obstructions of both carotid arteries," Dr. Gordon says. "After being told that the surgery being recommended for his condition is itself involved a high risk of stroke, he came to me. Since being placed on oral chelation therapy six years ago, he has had no further incidents of stroke".

Enzyme Therapy

In Germany, the Mucos Company has developed an all- natural combination enzyme-bioflavonoid product called Wobenzym-N that is widely available in most countries, including the U.S. Unlike most enzyme products on the market, this enzyme is specially designed not to digest food but to be used in the bloodstream to deal with many factors that can lead to cardiovascular conditions and other serious diseases, according to Dr. Gordon, including elevated fibrinogen and C-reactive protein. "This product provides all the benefits of anti-inflammatory medication without the high incidence of gastrointestinal bleeding and other side effects associated with long— term use of aspirin and NSAID," Dr. Gordon says.

Oxygen Therapy

Studies at Baylor University about 30 years ago found that an intravascular drip of hydrogen peroxide into leg arteries of atherosclerotic patients cleared arterial plaque. In cardiopulmonary resuscitations, hydrogen peroxide infusions often stopped ventricular fibrillation (rapid, ineffective contractions by the ventricles of the heart), the heart's response to insufficient oxygen.

The late Charles Farr, M.D., Ph.D., of Oklahoma City Oklahoma, reported success alternating treatments of IV. diluted hydrogen peroxide and chelation therapy to bring patients out of high-output heart failure (where the heart fails even though it is pumping a high amount of blood). Ozone therapy can also be used to treat arterial circulatory disturbances and to dissolve atherosclerotic plaque. Typically, injection of ozone into an artery is the method employed for this type of treatment.

Hyperbaric oxygen therapy (HBOT) is a form of oxygen therapy that is particularly effective as a treatment for stroke. "Every emergency room in the United States should have a hyperbaric oxygen chamber and every physician should be trained in its use," says David A. Steenblock, M.S., D.O., of Mission Viejo, California, a leading practitioner of HBOT for stroke. "If you can get more

195

oxygen to the brain within the first 24 hours of having a stroke, you can often salvage a great deal of brain tissue, eliminating 70% to 80% of the damage. Treating the patient by getting more oxygen to the brain during the first three weeks after the stroke makes it still possible to minimize the damage."

In fact, Dr. Steenblock has produced unexpected positive outcomes when treating people as long as 15 years after their stroke. The goal is to get as much oxygen into the brain as possible. This helps to revive oxygen-starved brain tissue that was damaged but not entirely destroyed when the stroke occurred.

Since 1971, over 1,000 cases demonstrating a 40% to 100% rate of improvement for stroke victims receiving HBOT have been reported in scientific journals.

Success Story: Eliminating the need for a Heart Transplant

As reported By Dr W Lee Cowden.

While conventional medicine often relies on the high- risk procedure of heart transplant in treating heart disease, this radical method can often be avoided.

Dr W. lee Cowden, M.D., of Fort Worth, Texas, reports the case of a 45-year-old physician who was suffering from pneumonia and an enlarged heart.

When given an ejection fraction test (measuring the percentage of the blood contained in the ventricle that is ejected on each heartbeat), his heart was only ejecting 16% of its contents (60% is normal), and his doctor told him his only hope was to receive a heart transplant. When he came into Dr Gowden's office, he could barely walk across the room with out becoming out of breath.

Dr. Cowden immediately put him on a detoxification program that included a vegetarian diet and a three-day vegetable juice fast with garlic He also had him follow a nutritional supplementation regimen including coenzyrne Q10, vitamin C, magnesium, vitamin complex, trace minerals, omega-3 fatty acids, lauric acid (an essential fatty acid), and carnitine, as well as the antiviral herbs St, John's Wort, Pfaffia paniculata, and Lomatium dissecturn.

Within three months, Dr. Cowden reports, the patient could jog ten miles a day and upon repeating the ejection fraction test, his score was up to 30%. Now he works 60 hours a week and continues to jog ten miles daily. **Source: Alternative Medicine:**

The Definitive Guide; Second Edition: Larry Trivieri, JR Editor, Introduced by Burton Goldberg

Non Western Medicine

Heart disease is not only a problem in Western countries. It is a global problem. Therefore remedies have been developed in the Chinese and Indian traditional medicine as well.

Traditional Chinese Medicine

Traditional Chinese medicine sees heart disease as a problem of poor digestion, which causes the buildup of plaque in the arteries.

Harvey Kaltsas,Ac.Phys. (FL), D.Ac. (RI), Dip.Ac. (NCCA) recommends herbs to strengthen digestive functioning. *"It has been understood in China for thousands of years that the circulation needs to flow unimpeded."*

He recommends a herbal extract from a plant known as mao-tung-ching (Ilex puibeceus) to dilate (widen) the blocked vessels. According to Dr. Kaitsas, it was proven in a Chinese study using mao-tung-ching four ounces orally or 20 mg intravenously on103 patients suffering from coronary heart disease that in 101 of the cases, there was significant improvement.

Dr Maoshing Ni, D.O.M., Ph.D., L.Ac., President of the Yo San University of Traditional Chinese Medicine, in Marina del Rey,

California, views heart disease as either a weakness or a block in the body's energy system.

For acute problems such as pain or abnormal heart rates, he uses acupuncture, but usually refers acute heart problem patients to a Western physician.

He says that Chinese Medicine is more suited to the treatment of chronic heart problems, for which he uses a combination of acupuncture and herbs to dissolve plaque, lower cholesterol levels, raise blood flow rates, and relieve angina.

One patient came to Dr. Ni after having an angioplasty because of 70% blockage of the coronary arteries. After the angioplasty, he still had 55% blockage. Dr. Ni treated him with herbs and acupuncture and, within four months, the blockage was reduced to 35%.

Ayurvedic Medicine

Ayurvedic practitioners use several methods that help with the reduction of the generation of free radicals, which can contribute to the disease process in the arteries and heart.

"Meat, cigarette smoke, alcohol, and environmental pollutants all generate free radicals," says Dr Han Sharma, M.D., F.R.C.P.C.,

Professor Emeritus of Ohio State University's College of Medicine and Public Health.

Dr. Sharma says: *"By using specific herbal food supplements and pancha karma (detoxification and purification) techniques, free radicals and lipid peroxides are reduced".*

Dr. Sharma also recommends a program of Transcendental Meditation to reduce stress. "As it is especially important for those with heart disease to lower their level of stress".

Virender Sodhi, M.D. (Ayurveda), N.D., Director of the Ayurvedic and Naturopathic Medical Clinic, in Bellevue, Washington, reports an interesting case of heart disease involving a 55-year-old Asian male with chest pain so severe that he could not walk more than ten steps before having to sit down.

He came to Dr. Sodhi's office after receiving word from the local hospital that he needed immediate bypass surgery. Refusing the surgery, doctors told him, would mean certain death.

Before beginning treatment, the man underwent a battery of tests ordered by Dr. Sodhi. Angiographic studies showed that the patient's coronary arteries were blocked—the left main coronary artery was only functioning by 10%, the anterior descending was functioning by 20%, and the right coronary was 30% blocked.

Blood tests indicated elevated cholesterol levels at 278 and decreased HDLs at 38. Dr. Sodhi determined his patient's metabolic type and started him on an appropriate cleansing program that included dietary changes and appropriate herbs.

After three months, the man's cholesterol levels reportedly dropped more than 30% and his HDLs rose to 48. More importantly, though, his exercise tolerance had dramatically improved. "He was doing the treadmill exercise," Dr. Sodhi reports, "at the speed of five miles per hour for 45 minutes without any angina." More than two years later, the patient was still doing fine, with improved EKG readings and able to jog up and down hills with no symptoms.

According to Dr.Sodhi, there is a hospital in Bombay, India, that has treated 3,300 cases of coronary heart disease using this method, with about 99% success.

Source: Alternative Medicine: The Definitive Guide; Second Edition: Larry Trivieri, JR Editor, Introduced by Burton Goldberg

Stress Reduction and Exercise

Stress has been called the big killer of our time. Stress is the factor that gets much of the blame for almost all of the serious diseases that we encounter these days. Not surprising then that reducing stress has therefore been proven to be highly effective in reversing heart disease.

In a study conducted by Dr. Ornish, an experimental group following a routine that combined a low-fat vegetarian diet, stress management, the elimination of smoking, and moderate exercise had a 91% decrease in the frequency of angina, as opposed to a control group that experienced a 165% increase in angina.

Control Aggression

A multinational study conducted in Canada, the U.S., and Israel, evaluated the effectiveness of an intervention aimed strictly at aggression reduction in patients with coronary artery disease. Participants learned listening skills to help reduce antagonism and techniques to avoid cynicism and anger. Patients who attended the full, eight-session course were observed to be less hostile and healthier than other patients. The study found the heart patients who released at least some of their aggression:

- Reduced their blood pressure

- Patients recovering from a heart attack saw a 50% reduction in subsequent rates of cardiac death.

Stress reduction can also play an important role in preventing heart disease Research showed that emotions such as anger, depression, and hopelessness can increase the likelihood of developing heart disease.

People with an angry temperament, who easily lose their temper at the slightest provocation, have been found to have nearly twice (200%) the risk of developing heart disease compared to people who get angry only when they have good cause, such as being unfairly treated or criticized.

Furthermore it was found that people who are angry and hostile also have higher levels of homocysteine, which increases heart disease risk.

Benefits of Exercise

Dr. Cowden includes stress-reduction exercises as part of his treatment. He believes that deep breathing and imaging techniques aimed at reducing stress should be conducted frequently throughout the day to reduce the output of stress hormones and lower the level of platelet aggregation. He encourages patients to do these techniques before meals and at bedtime, as they not only reduce stress but also can improve digestion. "The nutrients we are giving have to be absorbed out of the gastrointestinal tract. If the gut is in a stressed state, it will not absorb those nutrients nearly as well as if it is in a relaxed state."

Even ten minutes of extra exercise per day can significantly reduce the risk of heart disease – Dr W Lee Cowden, MD

Note: If you are in ill health or over the age of 40, check with your physician before beginning an exercise program.

It is also important for people with heart disease to get plenty of exercise, but many people have difficulty building a regular program of exercise into their lives.

David Essel, M.S., of Fort Myers Beach, Florida, provides some helpful tips to accomplish this:

- Move at least a little. Set a goal to walk, swim, skate, jump rope, aerobic dance, run, or ride a bike, three times a week for 20 minutes if possible, but even a ten-minute walk is better than nothing.

- Exercise can help you control or lose weight. This will likely have a positive effect on your cardiovascular health. Again, the amount of time you exercise is not the most important factor; that you exercise at all is what counts.

- Increasing lean muscle mass can improve your heart's health. A twice—weekly strength-training program using calisthenics, free weights, or exercise machines, in which the major muscle groups of the body (chest, back, legs, etc.) are exercised for up to three sets of 8-12 repetitions, can increase lean muscle tissue. This allows the body to burn more calories during the day, thereby assisting in weight loss.

- Keep to the program because exercise regularity is important. To stick with any program that enhances cardiovascular fitness, consider the following: invite a friend to exercise with you one or several days each week; schedule your exercise session in your daily planner so it has the same or higher priority as any other meeting for that day; or listen to your favorite music, book on tape, or motivational audio to inspire (or entertain) you during your workout.

A regular exercise program will reduce your blood pressure (if it was high), and you will also see a reduction in triglycerides and LDL cholesterol and an increase in HDL cholesterol.

Stopping a Heart Attack with your Hands!

Below is some life saving advice from Dr Glenn King Director of the King Institute for Better Health, in Dallas Texas,

According to Dr King, there are particular locations on your body called 'Energy Sphere Points," which, when you press gently on them with your fingers, can stop a heart attack or other serious conditions. King is the foremost U.S. practitioner of a little-known Asian health practice called Ki-iki-jutsu, which means "breath of life."

He describes it as "a finger-delivered form of therapy that allows the body, by its own tremendous power, to heal itself by un-constricting any stagnation or blockage of the natural energy circulatory patterns." Subtle bodily energy, known as qi or ki, flows along meridian pathways throughout the body, according to traditional Chinese medicine. By pressing certain pairs of points along the meridians, you can energetically, successfully treat seizures (as King experienced personally), heart attack, and other serious health conditions.

If you witness someone having a heart attack, place your right fingertips on the persons fifth thoracic vertebra (midway between

the most prominent parts of the shoulder blades on the back) and, with your other hand, hold the little finger of the person's left hand "This prompt action has consistently stopped heart attacks in progress," King states.

On average, this process can shift a person from being on the verge of entering cardiac arrest into a state of no sign of heart arrhythmia, pain, or discoloration within 24 minutes, King adds, noting that these results have been confirmed by cardiologists.

Source: Alternative Medicine: The Definitive Guide; Second Edition: Larry Trivieri, JR Editor, Introduced by Burton Goldberg

Recommended Reading

1. Alternative Cures: Bill Gottlieb

2. Alternative Medicine: The Definitive Guide; Second Edition: Larry Trivieri, JR Editor, Introduced by Burton Goldberg.

3. Natural Health A New Zealand A to Z Guide Lani Lopez

4. The Inflammation Syndrome – The Complete Nutritional Program to Prevent and Reverse Heart Disease, Arthritis, Diabetes, Allergies, Asthma. By Jack Challem

5. Encyclopedia of Natural Medicine Revised 2nd Edition : Michael Murray N.D. and Joseph Pizzorno N.D.

6. Alternative Medicine Guide to Heart Disease, Stroke & High Blood Pressure. Burton Goldberg and the Editors of Alternative Medicine. Tiburon, CA: Future Medicine Publishing, 1998.

7. Bypassing Bypass. Elmer Cranton. Charlottesville,VA: Hampton Roads Publishers, 2000.

8. Coping with Angina. Louise M.Wallace. London: Thor- sons, 1990.

9. Dr. Dean Ornish's Program for Reversing Heart Disease. Dean Ornish, M.D. NewYork: Ballantine, 1990.

10. Encyclopedia of Natural Medicine. Michael Murray, N.D., andJoseph Pizzorno, N.D. Rocklin, CA: Prima Publishing, 1998.

11. Good Cholesterol, Bad Cholesterol. Eli M. Roth, M.D., and Sandra L. Streicher, R.N. Rocklin, CA: Prima Publishing, 1993.

12. Heart Frauds: Uncovering the Biggest Health Scam in History. Charles T. McGee, M.D. Colorado Springs, GO: Health Wise Publications, 2001.

13. Heart Myths. Bruce D. Charash, M.D. NewYork:Viking Penguin, 1992.

14. The Johns Hopkins Complete Guide for Preventing and Reversing Heart Disease. Peter Kwiterovich, M.D. Rocidin, CA: Prima Publishing, 1998.

15. The New Supernutrition Book. Richard A. Passwater. New York: Pocket Books, 1991.

16. Plague Time: How Stealth Infections Cause Cancers, Heart Disease, and Other Deadly Ailments. Paul W. Ewald. New York: Free Press, 2000.

Acknowledgement of Scientists & Researchers

I have quoted extensively from the work of a large number of prominent scientists in the field of alternative health and wish to acknowledge them by this list.

- Dr Garry E Gordon, M.D., of Payson, Arizona, co-founder of the American College of Advancement in Medicine.

- Valentin Fuster, M.D., Ph.D., Director of the Cardiovascular Institute at Mount Sinai School of Medicine, in New York City.

- Dr James Privitera, M.D., of Covina, California.

- Paul W Ewald, Professor of Biology at Amherst College, author of the book Plague Time.

- Jack Challem author of "The Inflammation Syndrome" .

- Dr Philip Lee Miller, M.D., founder and director of the Los Gatos Longevity Institute in California.

- Dr Richard Passwater, Ph.D.

- Cardiologist Dr. W Lee Cowden, M. D.

- Dr Robert A. Anderson, M.D. founding President of the American Board of Holistic Medicine.

- Dr Broda O. Barnes, M.D., a Connecticut physician.

- Dr. Ichiro Kawachi of the Harvard School of Public Health.

- Cardiologist Dr Peter Langsjoen.

- Dr. Ravnskov author of the book The Cholesterol Myths.

- Nortin Hadler, M.D., Professor of Medicine at the University of North Carolina School of Medicine,

- American Heart Association by Henry Mcintosh, M.D.

- Dr Julian Whitaker, M.D. author of Reversing Heart Disease and founder and director of the Whitaker Wellness Institute in Newport Beach California.

- Dr Dean Ornish, M.D.,Assistant Clinical Professor of Medicine at the University of California at San Francisco.

- Michael Murray N.D. and Joseph Pizzorno N.D. authors of Encyclopedia of Natural Medicine Revised 2nd Edition:

- Amy Rothenberg, N.D., a naturopathic physician in Enfield, Connecticut.

- Mark Stengler, N.D., a naturopathic physician in San Diego.

- Kitty Gurkin Rosati, R.D., a registered dietitian and nutrition director of the Rice Diet Program at Duke University in Durham, North Carolina.

- Dr Matthias Rath, M.D., author of Eradicating Heart Disease, and former Director of the Linus Pauling Institute of Science and Medicine, in Palo Alto, California.

- Nobel laureate Dr Linus Pauling, Ph.D. and Dr Matthias Rath, M.D.

- Dr Philip Lee Miller, M.D., founder and director of the Los Gatos Longevity Institute in California.

- Dr. Abram Hoffer, M.D., Ph.D., of Victoria, British Columbia, Canada.

- Dr Moses M. Suzman, M.D., a South African neurologist and internist.

- Karl Folkers, Ph.D., a biomedical scientist at the University of Texas, in Austin.

- Researcher Dr Kilmer S. McCully, M.D.

- Researchers at Johns Hopkins University; in Baltimore, Maryland

- Dr. Alan R. Gaby, M.D., former President of the American Holistic Medical Association.

- David L. Hoffman, B.Sc., M.N.I.M.H., of Sebastopol, California, past President of the American Herbalists Guild.

- Dr Virender Sodhi, M.D. (Ayurved), N.D., an Ayurvedic and naturopathic physician and director of the American School of Ayurvedic Sciences in Bellevue, Washington.

- David L. Hoffman, B.Sc., M.N.I.M.H., of Sebastopol, California, past President of the American Herbalists Guild.

- David Hughes, Ph.D., of the Hyperbaric Oxygen institute, in San Bernardino, California.

- Harvey Bigelsen, M.D., Medical Director of the Center for Progressive Medicine, in Scottsdale, Arizona.

- Margaret A. Naeser, PhD., Associate Research Professor of Neurology at Boston University School of Medicine.

- David A. Steenblock, M.S., D.O., of Mission Viejo, California, a specialist in alternative treatments (especially hyperbaric oxygen) for stroke,

- Norman Clarke, Sr., M.D., Director of Research at Providence Hospital, in Detroit, Michigan.

- Efrain Olszewer, M.D., and James Carter, M.D., head of nutrition at the Department of Applied Health Science, School of Public Health and Tropical Medicine, at Tulane University.

- Charles Farr, M.D., Ph.D., of Oklahoma City Oklahoma.

- Harvey Kaltsas,Ac.Phys. (FL), D.Ac. (RI), Dip.Ac. (NCCA).

- Dr Maoshing Ni, D.O.M., Ph.D., L.Ac., President of the Yo San University of Traditional Chinese Medicine, in Marina del Rey, California.

- Dr Han Sharma, M.D., F.R.C.P.C., Professor Emeritus of Ohio State University's College of Medicine and Public Health.

- David Essel, M.S., of Fort Myers Beach, Florida.

- Dr. Patrick Quillin, R.D. Ph.D. director of the Rational Healing Institute in Tulsa, Oklahoma.

- Dr Stephen T. Sinatra, M.D., is a cardiologist and director of the New England Heart Center in Manchester, Connecticut.

- Dr Michael Janson, M.D., consultant physician at Path to Health in Burlington, Massachusetts.

- Dr Donald Carrow, M.D., founder and director of the Florida Institute of Health in Tampa.

More Books by John McArthur

Hypothyroidism
Hypothyroidism: The Hypothyroidism Solution. Hypothyroidism Natural Treatment and Hypothyroidism Diet for Under Active Or Slow Thyroid, Causing Weight Loss Problems, Fatigue, Cardiovascular Disease. John McArthur (Author), Cheri Merz (Editor)

Fibromyalgia And Chronic Fatigue
Fibromyalgia And Chronic Fatigue: A Step-By-Step Guide For Fibromyalgia Treatment And Chronic Fatigue Syndrome Treatment. Includes Fibromyalgia Diet And Chronic Fatigue Diet And Lifestyle Guidelines. John McArthur (Author), Cheri Merz (Editor)

Yeast Infection
Candida Albicans: Yeast Infection Treatment. Treat Yeast Infections With This Home Remedy. The Yeast Infection Cure. John McArthur (Author)

Heart Disease
Hypertension - High Blood Pressure: How To Lower Blood Pressure Permanently In 8 Weeks Or Less, The Hypertension Treatment, Diet and Solution. John McArthur (Author)

Cholesterol Myth: Lower Cholesterol Won't Stop Heart Disease. Healthy Cholesterol Will. Cholesterol Recipe Book & Cholesterol Diet. Lower Cholesterol Naturally Keep Cholesterol Healthy. John McArthur (Author), Cheri Merz (Editor)

Heart Disease Prevention and Reversal: How To Prevent, Cure and Reverse Heart Disease Naturally For A Healthy Heart. John McArthur (Author)

Diabetes
Diabetes Diet: Diabetes Management Options. Includes a Diabetes Diet Plan with Diabetic Meals and Natural Diabetes Food, Herbs and Supplements for Total Diabetes Control. Delicious Recipes. John McArthur (Author), Corinne Watson (Editor)

Diabetes Cooking: 93 Diabetes Recipes for Breakfast, Lunch, Dinner, Snacks and Smoothies. A Guide to Diabetes Foods to Help You Prepare Healthy Delicious ... Diabetic Meals and Natural Diabetes Food) John McArthur (Author), Corinne Watson (Editor)

Stress and Anxiety
From Stressful to Successful in 4 Easy Steps: Stress at Work? Stress in Relationship? Be Stress Free. End Stress and Anxiety. Excellent Stress Management, Stress Control and Stress Relief

Techniques. John McArthur (Author)

Anxiety and Panic Attacks: Anxiety Management. Anxiety Relief. The Natural And Drug Free Relief For Anxiety Attacks, Panic Attacks And Panic Disorder. John McArthur (Author), Cheri Merz (Editor)

Back and Neck Pain
The 15 Minute Back Pain and Neck Pain Management Program: Back Pain and Neck Pain Treatment and Relief 15 Minutes a Day No Surgery No Drugs. Effective, Quick and Lasting Back and Neck Pain Relief. John McArthur (Author)

Arthritis
Arthritis: Arthritis Relief for Osteoarthritis, Rheumatoid Arthritis, Gout, Psoriatic Arthritis, and Juvenile Arthritis. Follow The Arthritis Diet, Cure and Treatment Free Yourself From The Pain. John McArthur (Author)

Depression
How to Break the Grip of Depression: Read How Robert Declared War On Depression ... And Beat It! John McArthur (Author)

Pregnancy
Pregnancy Nutrition: Pregnancy Food. Pregnancy Recipes. Healthy Pregnancy Diet. Pregnancy Health. Pregnancy Eating and

Recipes. Nutritional Tips and 63 Delicious Recipes for Moms-to-Be. Corinne Watson (Author), John McArthur (Author)

Pregnancy and Childbirth: Expecting a Baby. Pregnancy Guide. Pregnancy What to Expect. Pregnancy Health. Pregnancy Eating and Recipes. Cheri Merz (Author), John McArthur (Author)

Allergies
Allergy Free: Fast Effective Drug-free Relief for Allergies. Allergy Diet. Allergy Treatments. Allergy Remedies. Natural Allergy Relief. John McArthur (Author), Cheri Merz (Editor)